OXFORD MEDICAL PUBLICATIONS

Blindness and visual handicap

THE FACTS

Blindness and visual handicap

THE FACTS

JOHN H. DOBREE

Consulting Ophthalmic Surgeon,
St. Bartholomew's Hospital, London

and

ERIC BOULTER

Former Director-General,
Royal National Institute for the Blind, London

OXFORD
OXFORD UNIVERSITY PRESS
NEW YORK TORONTO
1982

Oxford University Press, Walton Street, Oxford OX2 6DP

London Glasgow New York Toronto
Delhi Bombay Calcutta Madras Karachi
Kuala Lumpur Singapore Hong Kong Tokyo
Nairobi Dar es Salaam Cape Town
Melbourne Auckland

and associate companies in
Beirut Berlin Ibadan Mexico City

British Library Cataloguing in Publication Data
Dobree, John H.
Blindness and visual handicap. − (Oxford medical
publication)
1. Vision disorders
I. Title   II. Boulter, Eric
617.7'12   RE91
ISBN 0-19-261328-6

Library of Congress Cataloging in Publication Data
Dobree, John Hatherley.
Blindness and visual handicap.
(Oxford medical publications)
Bibliography: p.
Includes index.
1. Blind   2. Blindness.   I. Boulter, Eric,
1917-   .   II. Title.   III. Series.
HV1593.D6   362.4'18   82-3586
ISBN 0-19-261328-6   AACR2

Set by Hope Services, Abingdon
Printed in Great Britain by
Richard Clay (The Chaucer Press) Ltd,
Bungay, Suffolk.

Foreword

by

SIR JOHN WILSON C.B.E.,
Director, British Commonwealth Society for the Blind;
President, International Agency for the Prevention of Blindness

I was blinded by a school accident nearly 50 years ago. That accident must have changed the whole direction of my life but, looking back over those years, I am sure that it has not limited my opportunity or the zest and pleasure of living.

I had the good fortune to go to a fine school, Worcester College for the Blind. From there, on a scholarship, I went to Oxford University. I now have one of the most interesting jobs in the world, involving international travel and friendships in more than a hundred countries. I have a family life of great felicity. We have never been rich nor particularly wished to be but we have never been painfully poor. In all this I recognize great good fortune. Blindness can indeed be a disaster when compounded by loneliness, poverty, unemployment, and misunderstanding.

I remember the first time I saw a blind man. He was standing outside a shop door, a blank listening face behind dark obliterating spectacles. My swift reaction, as a seeing child, was a mixture of fear, pity, and a sense of strangeness. I have consciously preserved that memory. It has helped me to respect the anxiety of people who ask, not from curiosity but from real fear 'What would it be like if I went blind?' This book is written to help answer that question.

You could not have better guides to this world of blindness. John Dobree is an ophthalmic surgeon with an international standing in the field of medical ophthalmology. As Consultant Eye Surgeon to St. Bartholomew's Hospital for over twenty years he has had much experience of blinding diseases and of the way different individuals respond to the challenge of blindness. Eric Boulter is an outstanding international leader of work for the blind. In the course of a distinguished and varied career he has been Executive Head of the American Foundation for Overseas Blind (now Helen Keller International), Director-General of the Royal National Institute for the Blind, and President of the World Council for the Welfare of the Blind.

Acknowledgements

The authors acknowledge with thanks the valuable assistance extended by staff members of the Royal National Institute for the Blind and St. Dunstan's in the provision of resource material and photographs used in the preparation of this book. Our grateful thanks also go to Miss Charlotte McClure and Mrs Olive McDonald for their help in typing a considerable part of the text.

We also acknowledge with thanks our indebtedness to the following: Sir John Wilson for his helpful suggestions at the beginning of this work and for so kindly writing the Foreword; Mrs Jean Millard for all the original, distinct and artistic line-drawings; Dr John Marshall for his unique photographic studies of the retina and cornea; Mr W. D. Tredinnick of the Photographic Department, St. Bartholomew's Hospital for all the clinical studies and to Messrs Churchill Livingstone for permission to reproduce them from Birch's *Emergencies in medical practice*; Mr Richard Keeler for his helpful information on Low Vision Aids and for the plates illustrating them; the staff of Oxford University Press for much helpful editorial counsel.

London   J.H.D.
May 1982   E.B.

Contents

1

Introduction

This book has two authors: one of us is sighted and the other blind. Our aim has been to bring our two worlds closer together. The book is in two parts: the first deals with the diseases causing blindness and the second with the effects of blindness and the ways in which help can be given to the blind and partially sighted.

Part I describes the clinical aspects of eye disease. The emphasis is on conditions which may result in blindness and particularly those in which blindness is preventable. It is based on lectures given to many generations of medical students and student nurses at St. Bartholomew's Hospital so it is hoped that the reader will forgive a certain lack of formality or an occasional irrelevancy.

We hope that the book may be useful to medical practitioners, nurses, opticians, welfare workers, and others who come into contact with the blind and partially sighted in the course of their professional work. Above all we hope that it may be intelligible to entirely non-medical people: those perhaps who fear loss of sight themselves or in someone close to them and who would like to learn a little more about eye diseases. To this end a glossary of medical terms has been appended.

The second part of the book describes the effects of blindness whether it occurs in the old, the young, or those in the prime of life. There are varying degrees of blindness and in the way it strikes. Sometimes, as with battle casualties, it is swift and final; sometimes slow and insidious, as it is in chronic glaucoma. Again there is a difference between the blindness of those who have never seen at all and those who have a vivid visual memory. All this means that there are many ways in which people react to their blindness and how they come to terms with it. It is for this reason we have included some biographical studies of blind people from Homer to recent times.

The final chapters deal with the way in which the blind and partially sighted can be helped. In most countries state social services and voluntary organizations have this as their prime purpose. A necessary step to obtain benefits in the United Kingdom is Blind Registration. This registration is described in some detail as there are often misconceptions about it. It does not mean, for example, that doctors have given up hope. It ensures that, apart from coming under the protective wing of the state, the patient has a thorough examination by a consultant ophthalmologist so that any optical aids or surgery which may improve the vision can be offered.

Then there are practical aids to enable the blind to keep their independence. How does one obtain a talking book — or a guide dog? What gadgets are available for the housewife? What are low vision aids and how are they obtained? How and where can one be trained in the use of the 'long cane'? These and many other questions are answered.

Some of the problems of the education of the blind are considered too. The method of educating a blind child is a controversial issue. Are the visually handicapped better able to take their place in the world if they have been integrated in an ordinary school at an early age or should they be educated in special schools?

Then there are those who lose their sight during their working life. Some can continue with their jobs as before but most need rehabilitation and retraining for other jobs. How is this done — and where?

The last chapter of the book is a very important one: what practical help can the sighted individual give to the blind? There is a wealth of concern towards the blind but how can it be most effectively channelled? We meet blind people in differing circumstances: sometimes as a relative or close friend in daily or hourly contact; sometimes as an occasional visitor, and sometimes as total strangers in brief encounters. This chapter gives guidelines on when the blind are likely to need help, and how it can best be given, and how the worlds of the blind and the sighted can be brought closer together.

Part I

Causes of blindness

JOHN H. DOBREE

2

The anatomists and the eye

Ophthalmology is the study of the eye; its functions and diseases. The anatomy of the eye is part of that study, and a fascinating one too. It is important because without a knowledge of the normal structure of the eye, which is precisely what anatomy is about, we cannot hope to know how the parts differ in disease states: the pathology of the eye. Moreover, if we do not understand the pathology of any eye disease there is little hope of its effective treatment.

The early civilizations

The recorded history of ophthalmology goes back to ancient Babylon. In the hot, dry, and dusty lands of the Middle East the exposed parts of the eyes suffer from a multitude of diseases; the external eye diseases: diseases of the lids such as styes, cysts, or ingrowing eyelashes which abrade the cornea, the transparent window of the eye (Fig. 1) or inflammations of the conjunctiva, the membrane which lines the back of

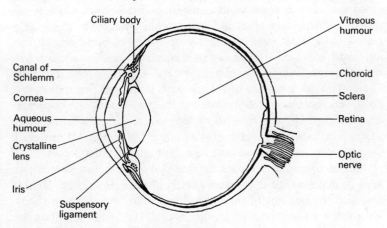

Fig. 1. Vertical section through eyeball.

the lids. All these conditions, many of them blinding, were recorded by the Babylonians and ancient Egyptians, who gave some very practical advice on their treatment.

It is possible that these early peoples knew of conditions inside the eye too but we have no proof of this. Medicine was in the hands of the priests and if surgery was performed it was under their direction by a lower order of skilled hand-workers. There were also technical difficulties. The delicate structures of the eye demand very fine and sharp instruments for dissection and surgery; far finer than the knives of bronze and obsidian which were then in use.

The Greeks and Romans

Mankind had to wait 1500 years, for the age of Hippocrates (460–377 BC), before medicine freed itself from the shackles of religion, and the old order of priestcraft and the supernatural were finally abandoned. The Greeks began to observe and to think afresh. Among the important observations they made were those on the anatomy of the eye.

Aristotle of Athens (384–322 BC) dissected the eyes of apes and other animals and concluded rightly that the eyeball is essentially a sphere composed of three concentric layers. These are the three coats we know today (see Fig. 1). There is an outer tough protective layer called the sclera because of its hardness, and the cornea which is the smaller front portion of it, no less tough but transparent. The middle coat is the choroid, which is mainly composed of blood-vessels. The innermost coat is the retina, a thin transparent membrane which was not until centuries later recognized for the all-important tissue that it is. The curtain-like structure of the iris with its central perforation, the pupil, was also known to Aristotle but there was considerable speculation at this period as to why the pupil appeared black. On cutting open an eye one finds in the centre no black object but transparent matter of varying consistency. This was an enigma not solved by the Greeks.

The art of medicine eventually died slowly in ancient Greece but lived on in Alexandria in the century after Christ. Celsus (25 BC–50 AD) described the anatomy of the eye and was aware that the ciliary body and the iris are continuous with the choroid. He further described the crystalline lens, also known as the crystalline humour, which is the most obvious of the central transparent parts of the eye. Another anatomist of this school, Rufus of Ephesus (c. AD 100) recognized three humours. Between the front of the lens and the cornea he found a watery fluid he called the aqueous humour. Behind the lens, between it and the retina, he described a jelly-like substance rather the consistency of egg-white, which he knew as the vitreous humour. Between these two humours was the third, the lens itself, or crystalline humour.

The Greek tradition of medicine passed from Alexandria to Rome and the greatest figure to emerge from this period is that of Galen (131–210) state physician to the Emperor Marcus Aurelius. His theories of medicine were accepted until the Middle Ages of Europe. Galen recognized the ciliary body but had no notion of its function any more than he had of that of the transparent humours. Indeed, in his time the crystalline lens, because of its position near the centre of the globe, was credited with being the actual organ of sight. Although Galen recognized the optic nerve or 'stalk' of the eye and knew of its connection with the nerve from the other eye and even of the crossing or 'chiasma' below the brain, it was not realized that the actual seat of vision is in a small area of the hindermost part of the brain: the occipital cortex.

The Renaissance

After Galen little was added to the knowledge of the anatomy of the eye until the Renaissance, and then it was not the doctors who led the way but the artists. Their careful studies of the human form demanded a knowledge of muscle, bone, and blood-vessels below the surface. And get that knowledge they would, despite the proscription on dissection of the human body by Mother Church. Among her least obedient sons was Leonardo da Vinci, who claimed to have dissected thirty bodies. He knew of the camera obscura, the device whereby in a darkened chamber, a bright panoramic view of the world outside can be projected on a screen, and he recognized the similarity of the optics of the camera obscura to those of the eye.

In the sixteenth and seventeenth centuries the great universities of Europe and schools of medicine provided intellectual havens where men could study and ideas become disseminated. The great anatomist Fallopius of Padua (1523-62), who gave his name to the tubes of the oviduct, also described the capsule of the crystalline lens, which we shall meet again in the study of cataract. Later Ruysch (1638–1731) described the muscles of the iris, the action of which regulates the size of the pupil.

Van Leeuwenhoek: the microscope

There is a limit to the detail the human eye can see even with the aid of a magnifying lens but one singularly pertinacious Dutchman brought about a momentous advance. This was Anthony van Leeuwenhoek (1632–1723), a draper from Delft. He was a man of no scientific knowledge or training, spoke only his native Dutch, and had no knowledge of Latin which was the accepted language of the scientists of the day. Leeuwenhoek had one ruling passion in life: the making of microscopes. He ground and polished his own lenses and built up the metalwork of innumerable microscopes, each one able to show up more detail than the last. Then with them he explored a new world: a world never before seen by man.

He was a most accurate and honest observer and he drew everything he saw in a wide variety of subjects: the sting of a bee, for example, or animalcules in a drop of water from his water-butt. Of the human tissues he examined he was the first to see the cells in the blood, and a spermatozoon (his own, in fact, for which he made due apology to the gentlemen of the Royal Society of England to whom he was in the habit of reporting his discoveries). In the eye he saw the fibrils of which the crystalline lens is composed and also the rods and cones of the retina, the little torpedo-shaped sense organs by which we perceive light impulses. But like so many other innovators Leeuwenhoek was before his time and many of his observations had to wait half a century or more for confirmation; but the Dutchman was always proved right!

After Leeuwenhoek's death the microscope became more and more widely used as a scientific instrument and the microscopists learned the technique of cutting thin sections of tissue embedded in wax and staining them with dyes which revealed the structure of the cells of which all living tissue is composed. Later, with increasing magnification, it was possible to see minute details of the cells themselves and how they alter in disease.

8

The anatomists and the eye

One of the greatest observers of this era of microscopists was an Englishman, William Bowman (1812–92). As a young man he made a series of brilliant discoveries on the minute anatomy of the kidney and later, the eye. He identified five layers of tissue in the cornea and one of them (Bowman's membrane) still carries his name. Bowman was a prodigious worker and, despite the fact that he had a flourishing London practice and became Sir William and the Queen's oculist, he continued his scientific work to the end of his life.

Helmholtz: the ophthalmoscope

One cannot see into the interior of the eye because of the reflections from the cornea. The difficulty was overcome a little over a century ago by a young German scientist, Hermann von Helmholtz. He invented an instrument he called the 'eye mirror'. Light was reflected into the eye by the mirror and the observer, looking along the light from behind, obtained a clear view of the interior of the eye, or the fundus as it is usually called. Later, when a hole in the mirror was used for viewing, and by adding a series of lenses to bring any part into focus, the modern ophthalmoscope was born.

The fundus so revealed is shown in Fig. 2. It is in fact seen in brilliant colour. The most striking feature is the optic disc or commencement of the optic nerve with the retinal vessels radiating from it. The macula, situated a little to the outer side, is the place where we have our most acute vision for form and colour.

It is in conditions of disease that the oculist finds the ophthalmoscope his greatest boon. We can see *living* pathology, about twenty times magnified. We shall see that many of the eye diseases have distinctive fundus appearances. Furthermore many of the general bodily diseases such as diabetes, raised blood-pressure, blood diseases, diseases of the nervous system, and many others can be seen through the window of the eye more clearly than by any other means.

Later in his life, Helmholtz described the means whereby the eye can focus both on near and distant objects. He showed that the tiny muscles in the ciliary body are able to exert a pull on the fibres of the suspensory ligament of the lens and so alter its curvature.

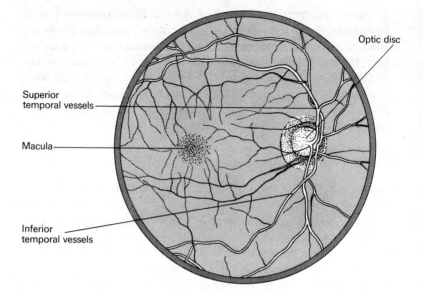

Optic disc

Superior
temporal vessels

Macula

Inferior
temporal vessels

Fig. 2. Ophthalmoscope view of right fundus

Recent discoveries

There is always a tendency to think that we have reached the ultimate
discovery, and yet each time the horizon retreats again. After the light
microscope had yielded many secrets of the eye the electron microscope
was developed, which can 'blow-up' a single cell to the size of this page
or much larger. Thus the smallest details of individual cells and their
surrounding membranes are revealed. Then there is the scanning electron
microscope which allows three-dimensional pictures to be made, and
these show additional features.

It is also possible by means of closed-circuit television to study the
blood-flow in the living eye. And even when one cannot see into the
eye because the transparent parts have become opaque it is still possible
by means of ultrasound techniques to get an accurate picture of the
structures in the interior of the eye.

The anatomists and the eye

The discoveries of the anatomists have served to tell us about the basic anatomy of the eye. When we come to consider conditions such as cataract and glaucoma we shall add some additional anatomical facts which relate both to the diseases and their treatment.

3

Disorders of the retina

The retina is the key structure of the eye. If the retina fails the eye is blind; if there is some retinal response — even a faint glimmer of light — the possibility of worthwhile sight exists.

The retina is really an extension of the brain but set forward from it the better to gather information. A picture of the outside world is actually formed on the retina and transmitted by the optic nerve to the brain. In the brain the picture is interpreted and then stored in the memory.

Anatomy

The retina is composed of nerve tissue. It is about as thick as a piece of blotting paper and as easy to tear as when that paper is wet. It is perfectly transparent apart from the columns of blood in its own system of blood-vessels. It also has a second blood-supply from the very rich circulation of the choroid which surrounds it.

Under the microscope (Plate 1) the retina is seen to consist of ten layers of tissue lying like the pages of a book. Only the nerve cells are showing and not the labyrinth of nerve fibres which connect them. The outermost layer, nearest the choroid, is highly specialized tissue called the pigment cell layer and is described on p. 20. The other nine layers are neural tissue. The layer adjacent to the pigment cell layer is the layer of rods and cones and is concerned with the reception of light impulses. The remaining eight layers, the transmitting layers, are concerned with sending the impulses to the brain by the optic nerve.

Function

The retina can be likened to a telephone exchange in which each subscriber is able to make local or trunk calls and so gather information from a wide area. It can also do the equivalent of photographing and developing a colour film every tenth of a second throughout all the waking hours. For this it needs an abundant supply of oxygen. But the analogy of the retina to a camera film ends here, for there is a striking difference. Whereas a camera film is manufactured to ensure that all parts of the film are equally sensitive, the retina is designed so that the central part is much more sensitive than the peripheral areas. This is due to the different functions of cells called the rods and cones.

The cones are nerve cells shaped like little rockets (Plate 1) with the pointed ends facing forward. They are most numerous in the macula area, where they greatly outnumber the rods. In fact in the centre of the macula is a small area called the fovea which is entirely composed of cones. Cones are sensitive to minute detail and to colour and so are responsible for the most acute vision. The rods are cigar-shaped cells (Plate 1). They are sensitive to movement and are used particularly in conditions of semi-darkness (twilight vision). The rods are most numerous in the peripheral parts of the retina and are more sparsely distributed in the central areas. Before we discuss the way these two cell types work together, it is necessary to know something about the visual fields.

The visual field of each eye is the whole panorama which can be seen surrounding the object (the fixation spot) which one is looking at. The inner (nasal) portions of the visual fields overlap and the outer (temporal) fields allow us to see directly sideways to the left and right. If you stretch out one arm and extend the fingers the area covered by the palm is roughly the size of the area served by the macula; away from this the vision drops off sharply towards the periphery. There are therefore two elements to a visual field: a central and a peripheral and the way they are linked may be illustrated in the following way.

Imagine one of our prehistoric ancestors on a hunting expedition. He is hungry and night is falling. His eyes scan the landscape. He cannot possibly take in every detail of what is there but there are certain things that he cannot afford to miss. For example, there is a slight movement in a group of saplings some fifty paces to his right. This movement is picked up by the rod cells of his peripheral retina. What is it? Another man? – an enemy perhaps? An animal he can kill? – or just a small bird settling down to roost? Without conscious effort he brings both his eyes to bear on the area of interest and the cones of his macular areas start

13

to give his brain much more detailed information as to what is happening there. It was the movement of the head of a deer, its shape now clearly visible between the branches and the ruddy colouring of its neck confirming it. But it is already away. Later, darkness falls and the only light comes from a crescent moon. Our hunter is now relying entirely on the rods of the peripheral parts of his retinae and has no vision from the cones in his macular areas. He sees a world without colour and little detail but he is able to get about and may yet catch that deer asleep!

In health then the two parts of the retina work as a team: the peripheral retina supplies the broad outline and the macula the detail. There are many causes of retinal blindness. In some the macula bears the brunt of the disease and in others the periphery is at fault. Sometimes the whole retina is involved. Let us study the more important of these conditions.

Diabetic retinopathy

For many people their work is their life and in Europe and North America the eye condition most likely to enforce early retirement is diabetic eye disease. Often both eyes are affected and it accounts for some 12 per cent of all blind registrations under the age of 65. Concepts about the nature of diabetes are changing rapidly. What was formerly considered to be a condition in which sugar could not be properly used by the body is now recognized to be much more complex. In particular it is now known that there is widespread damage to the walls of many of the blood-vessels of the body, including those of the retina.

There are two forms of diabetic retinopathy and these often occur together. People who develop diabetes before the age of 15 are called juvenile diabetics and they are dependent on insulin to keep well. At some time before the age of 40 they may develop a condition called proliferative retinopathy. This is characterized by the formation of 'new-formed' blood-vessels which sprout from the normal retinal vessels; they are very thin-walled and liable to bleed. On the other hand those who develop diabetes in middle life are known as maturity-onset diabetics. These people suffer from damage to capillary blood-vessels, particularly in the region of the posterior pole. This leads to deposits of fatty material (lipoid exudates) in the retina and the formation of small pin-point haemorrhages. This condition is called simple (or exudative) retinopathy and runs a slower and more benign course.

Proliferative retinopathy

The new vessels which slowly develop from the pre-existing normal retinal arteries and veins have very thin walls and are very liable to rupture and cause haemorrhages inside the eye. Sometimes these bleedings are small and pass unnoticed by the patient. If however they are large the blood runs into the vitreous gel and a rapid loss of vision occurs: this can be an alarming experience. The patient sees the moving shadows of the blood cells like a swarm of bees and if the haemorrhage is large the vision becomes more and more hazy for the next few minutes until it may be reduced to perception of light and take weeks or months to clear again. Further, permanent damage may be done to the retina for the clot may condense and form opaque curtain-like structures in the vitreous, or bands of tissue which may subsequently contract and detach the retina.

But this is painting a rather gloomy picture: the vast majority of vitreous haemorrhages clear in a few days to a few weeks and leave no aftermath. The trouble is, however, that they are apt to recur. To a large extent they can be avoided, as the factor which causes a vessel to break is a physical strain of the type which causes congestion of the blood-vessels of the head. These strains are mostly avoidable and include many domestic chores such as moving furniture, lifting heavy weights, and scrubbing floors. Furthermore strains such as a paroxysm of coughing, vomiting, or constipation can easily cause a rupture of these delicate new vessels. There is however no need to wrap the patient up in cotton-wool. Exercise such as walking or swimming is not harmful nor is normal sexual intercourse. If a haemorrhage does occur the best first-aid treatment is to go straight to bed with the head resting comfortably.

In recent years the outlook for cases of proliferative diabetic retinopathy has been much improved by the advent of light (photo-) coagulation to the new vessels and by surgery. Light coagulation is a powerful beam of light from a xenon arc or argon laser directed on to an area of damage which one wishes to eradicate. The exact spot is selected by an ophthalmoscope with a sighting beam and when the full strength of the laser beam is turned on, a localized white patch, the burn, is formed. The transparent media of the eye are unaffected by the light and the burn is formed only where there are pigmented cells such as those in the retinal pigment layer (see p. 20).

Surgery is used in the later stages of proliferative retinopathy: using delicate cutting instruments to remove opaque bands and membranes or cutting out the whole of the vitreous when this is filled with persistent clot (Vitrectomy) (see p. 37).

Simple diabetic retinopathy

Simple (or exudative) retinopathy differs from proliferative retinopathy in several respects. Not only are the pathological changes more likely to be found in middle life and after but the damage they cause takes much longer to develop. In simple retinopathy the essential fault is a weakening or breaking of the walls of some of the capillaries, particularly those in the posterior pole just to the outer side of the macula.

The earliest sign of impending trouble is the appearance of micro-aneurysms. These appear as minute red dots on ophthalmoscopy and they are caused by bulging of the weakened capillary walls. Some capillaries actually break and form small retinal haemorrhages. At the same time plasma escapes from them and causes an oedema (waterlogging) of the neighbouring retina. With the plasma come fatty substances which normally circulate in the bloodstream. These are called lipoids and they slowly, over months or years, become deposited in the outer plexiform layer of the retina. They often form a ring around the damaged capillaries and are called 'hard' exudates. If they form at the macula, which is not unusual, they interfere with vision.

The best way of studying the circulation of the retina is by means of a technique called fluorescein angiography. Fluorescein dye is injected into a vein and passes into the circulation. When it arrives at the retina it is photographed using a blue light which shows up in great detail all blood-vessels, down to the smallest capillaries. It also shows where the capillaries are damaged and leaking. These places are noted and subjected later to light coagulation which causes a scar and seals them up. The hard exudates disappear after a few months and the retinal oedema subsides.

It is important that diabetics should have their blood sugar well controlled by insulin or antidiabetic tablets. If there are any signs of retinopathy a six-monthly check is made to ensure that no new vessels or macular exudates are forming. Diabetic cataract is discussed on p. 40.

Macular degeneration

In general the more highly developed a tissue is the more vulnerable it is likely to be. The macula is no exception to this rule; many disease conditions strike here and when they do the vision is seriously affected. The most common of these macular disorders is a condition called macular degeneration, or 'senile' degeneration because it is mostly found in the over-sixties. It is caused by a defective blood-supply to the macula.

The macula gets the larger part of its blood-supply from the capillary blood-vessels of the choroid. In younger people these capillaries ensure that a liberal supply of oxygen is available, but as a person becomes older some capillaries become narrowed and some close down entirely. Others start to leak; the fluid part of the blood (plasma) escapes first but if the leakage is more severe an actual haemorrhage occurs. Again 'new vessels' may form from the surviving choroidal capillaries and these again may leak and bleed. All this means that the ophthalmoscopic appearances are very variable, depending on whether one is seeing the result of leakage or changes in the retina secondary to oxygen lack. The result however is the same: a marked loss of vision for detail and for colour.

When one loses macular vision the very thing that one wants to look at simply disappears. This is called a central scotoma or shadow. One gets the best result by looking a little to the side of whatever it is one wants to see and so avoiding the blank spot. But even quite close to the macula the retina is nothing like so sensitive as the macula itself and only a very poor image can be obtained. A typical case-history illustrates the slow progress of the condition.

Five years ago: Mrs A has recently noticed that when she covers up the left eye and uses the right eye alone the letters of the word that she is actually reading appear to be distorted. Certain familiar outlines which she knows perfectly well should be straight, like her picture rail or the mantle shelf, are kinked. With the left eye everything is perfectly normal.

Blindness and visual handicap: the facts

Three years ago: The vision in the right eye is now considerably worse. She can read headlines with the right eye but there is a blur centred on the very object she wants to see. The left eye too has now become a bit blurred but she can just see to read with it. However, she has to use a magnifying glass for telephone numbers.

Two years ago: She is now having difficulty with anything requiring detailed vision with either eye. She has had to give up her fine sewing and tapestry but can still do the essential mending and darning. She gave up her morning paper last year but was able to read 'large-print' books from the library until quite recently. With the help of a magnifying lens she can make out essential things like the amount on a cheque. She can even read letters from her daughter who knows about her difficulty and writes large with a felt pen. She is still able to enjoy television especially since her son gave her a colour set but cannot make out any of the credits or captions.

This year: She now pays annual visits to her eye doctor. He checks that there is no sign of cataract or glaucoma as these conditions affect the elderly and might need treatment. This time she notices that she is only able to see the top letter of the test types with each eye. She gets very depressed at this but the surgeon surprisingly enough is reassuring up to a point, and tells her that although the condition may get a little worse in the next few years she will be able to manage most things without help. This is a huge relief: Mrs A has dreaded that she is going to go completely blind, lose her independence, and 'be a burden on people'. However, although the vision for detail will be lost the part of the retina used for getting about will not be affected. She will see quite enough to get around by herself and to see things like where the electric light switch and lavatory handle are situated, even in another person's house.

It is at about this stage that the doctor would send Mrs A to a Low Vision Aid Centre, as there are several optical appliances that may help her. Simply giving her stronger glasses probably would not help very much as there is a limit to the magnification that can be obtained with glasses (see p. 182). He would probably also put her name on the Partially-sighted Register (see p. 129).

This case history is very typical: it shows the slow development of the condition and how only the central vision is affected. The outlook must be carefully explained to the patient at the outset as they are fully aware that the vision is deteriorating and fear that they will become completely blind.

It is only rarely possible to treat cases of macular degeneration as one is dealing with what is essentially part of the aging process. There is no scientifically established medical treatment but occasionally in selected cases in which the new vessels come from the choroidal circulation and are causing oedema in the overlying retina, the condition can be improved by very careful laser treatment.

Retinitis pigmentosa (see also p. 91).

Retinitis pigmentosa, in which the peripheral parts of the retina bear the brunt of the degenerative condition, is the most common of a group of conditions called abiotrophies in which the retinae of both eyes are affected. It gets its name from the fact that its appearance with the ophthalmoscope is very typical; there are little clumps of pigment strewn over the fundus rather like seaweed on the sea shore. It has a strong tendency to run in families but isolated cases often occur. In childhood the patient seems to see perfectly well but later, usually some time between the age of 5 and 20, difficulties arise. The most obvious of these is defective vision in reduced light, often called night blindness.

In absolute darkness even an owl cannot see but under even very reduced illumination (starlight for example) a normal person gradually becomes more and more used to the poor light so that in about half an hour like our hunter in the introduction to this chapter he sees enough to get about. We say then that he is dark adapted. There is no appreciation of colour but he sees outlines and movements clearly. Now what happens when our dark-adapted person suddenly enters a well-lit room? There is immediately a blinding glare but he rapidly gets used to the light and in about 30 seconds he sees detail and colour as before; we say now he is light-adapted. In retinitis pigmentosa the light adaptation is normal but the dark adaptation is defective.

In families in which cases of retinitis pigmentosa occur the diagnosis is usually made early as it is anticipated; indeed it can be made in the early months of life by the use of electronic testing. Usually it is the difficulty in getting about in semi-darkness that brings other cases to attention.

The condition is progressive although the visual acuity and colour vision are normal. The peripheral field of vision becomes gradually more and more reduced until after a number of years the patient has 'tunnel-vision'. This means that there is a brilliantly clear central field of 10-20° and surrounding this, darkness. The patient now has difficulty in getting about in daylight as he keeps knocking into things and has to be constantly on guard whenever moving about. Sometimes the field loss stops in its tracks for an indefinite period but the more usual course is relentless progression. Vision is usually retained until middle life. Not infrequently a central secondary cataract adds to the difficulties.

Patients with retinitis pigmentosa do well at jobs in which there is little moving about involved and for which fine detail is needed. Occupations such as making jewellery, watch-repairing, or electronic assembly are ideal for these people.

The condition is always present in much the same degree in both eyes. Many cases are familial: in some families there are numerous cases which occur in every generation (dominant inheritance) and in some the cases crop up sporadically in the family tree with some generations escaping entirely (recessive inheritance). In some again the condition is transmitted by mothers who have normal vision but who transmit the condition to their male offspring (sex-linked inheritance).

Where there is a known genetic defect like retinitis pigmentosa in a family, a couple considering having children should avail themselves of genetic counselling. This is a job for specialists and outside the scope of this book. The advice given as to the risk of children having the condition transmitted to them depends on factors such as any blood relationship between the couple, whether or not there are cases of retinitis pigmentosa on both sides, and how many generations have been affected. Genetic counselling is available at an increasing number of centres and those wishing to use them should, in the first instance, consult their general practitioners and obtain referral through them. See also retinitis pigmentosa in children (p. 91).

Retinal detachment

We have seen that the retina consists of ten layers. The front nine layers are made entirely of nerve tissue and closely connected to each other by nerve fibrils. The back layer however is quite unlike the others. It is called the pigment cell layer. It is composed of a single layer of rather squat cells which contain granules of a brown pigment. These pigment cells carry out several important functions. Among them are the proper functioning of the rods and cones.

There is no direct continuity between the pigment layer and the rods and cones; the two layers are simply pressed together. They are easily separated by intra-ocular fluid (p. 50), and when this happens a detachment of the retina is said to be present.

Types of retinal detachment

There are several different types of retinal detachment. The most common is the so-called rhegmatogenous detachment. This is preceded by a hole or tear in the neural layers of the retina which allows the intra-ocular fluid to percolate through the gap and to strip the neural layers of the retina away from the pigment cell layer. If the condition is untreated, the detachment slowly increases over the next few days or weeks until it is complete. Any part of the retina which is detached is separated from its choroidal blood-supply and becomes blind. If however the condition is treated by sealing the hole the fluid absorbs, the neural layers of the retina fall back into place, and the rods and cones link up with the pigment cells once more. Vision is then restored.

Another way in which a retinal detachment occurs is by so-called traction detachment; this is very common in diabetic retinopathy. It will be remembered that the new vessels and the bleeding which accompanies them cause connective tissue bands to form inside the eye. These bands slowly contract and as this happens the layers of the retina are gradually pulled apart. There are not usually any holes in the retina in cases of traction detachments, and the tenting effect on the retina often stays stationary for months or years without causing much loss of vision, unless the macula is involved. A third type of detachment is associated with a malignant melanoma of the choroid (p. 49).

Causes

How do retinal holes form in the first place? There are several possible causes. Unlike some body tissues such as tendon, which is as strong as nylon, the retina has little tensile strength: it is more like brain tissue of which it is a forward extension. Retinal holes often occur following a blow on or near the eye and many boxers suffer retinal detachments

(p. 64). A very myopic (short-sighted) person may have a weak retina due to the expansion of the globe in this condition. Many detachments occur in middle life and after; these are usually due to a weakening of the retina caused by degeneration of the blood-vessels of the retina and choroid. Detachments are also common after cataract extraction (aphakic detachment) and associated with melanoma of the choroid (p. 49).

Symptoms

A detachment of the retina may give rise to distinctive symptoms. For example there is sometimes a sensation as though a small electric bulb is flashing on and off in some part of the visual field. This denotes some disturbance to the retina which has only one response to stimuli, that of the sensation of light. In this case it is possible that the retina is tearing; this is even more likely if the flashes are associated with an impression that the room is filled with a swarm of bees. This sensation is caused by the patient's red blood cells escaping into the vitreous and forming visible 'floaters' (p. 37). The two symptoms are linked because the tear of the retina may also rupture some of the retinal capillary blood-vessels and thereby produce a haemorrhage.

These symptoms of 'flashes' and 'swarms of bees' are important because they form an 'early-warning' system that something is amiss. The same symptoms are also found in other fundus diseases such as retraction of the vitreous which is a benign disorder. But the wise oculist makes a particularly careful search of the retina should they be reported. There is a sound reason for this. The holes or tears which give rise to the symptoms are 'flat' in the early stages; that is the intra-ocular fluid has not at this stage percolated through the hole and the retina has not yet become detached. But this state of affairs is not going to remain indefinitely. In a matter of days a retinal detachment may start to form. At the 'flat hole' stage it is a relatively simple matter to seal off the hole (p. 23) by light coagulation or cryotherapy but if fluid has started to collect major surgery will be needed to treat the detachment.

When the retina does detach the collection of subretinal fluid increases and the retina is thrown into folds. Wherever the detachment is present the retina is blind, so the patient may notice a gradual reduction of the visual field which corresponds to the collection of fluid; bearing in mind of course that the retinal projection is inverted so that a collection of subretinal fluid below will give a defect in the upper field.

In an untreated case the detachment and the field loss gradually increase and there is a marked loss of vision if the macula becomes involved. The condition usually passes into the final stage when the detachment becomes complete and the eye is blind.

Treatment

Until some fifty years ago retinal detachment was an incurable condition but improvements in the diagnostic examination and especially in the identification of holes has lead to a high percentage of cures, about 80 per cent of cases now recover vision. Some cases, however, are not amenable to treatment and as the condition often occurs in both eyes blindness sometimes follows.

If a flat hole of the retina exists it is usually quite easy to treat by surrounding it with a ring or double ring of 'burns' by means of photocoagulation under direct vision or by application of a freezing probe (cryopexy) to the sclera overlying the hole. In both cases an aseptic inflammation is set up in the choroid and as this heals the retina and choroid adhere firmly to each other and make a permanent seal around the hole.

If a true retinal detachment is present with separation of the neural and pigment cell layers by subretinal fluid much more elaborate techniques are required to rectify the condition. The first essential is to make a careful examination of the retina to make sure that all the holes have been located. These are then carefully marked out on a chart which enables all the holes or suspect areas to be projected on to the surface of the sclera. Great experience and care are necessary to achieve this. Just as for flat holes, the sclera overlying the raised holes is subjected to cryopexy (freezing) or diathermy (heat) and the subsequent inflammation causes the retina and choriod to adhere. In some cases the union is made easier by indenting the sclera by means of a small plastic sponge and in others by encircling the equator of the globe by a plastic strap. Both sponge and strap cause the subretinal fluid to absorb more easily and sometimes it is necessary to 'tap' off some of the fluid by a small hollow tube (cannula).

23

In cases of traction detachment the bands which cause the condition are sometimes best left alone as the detachment may remain localized. At other times, especially if the macula is threatened, they respond to encirclement or by surgical division of the bands.

Retinal vascular diseases

We already know that the retina has a double blood-supply: first its own system, the four major retinal arteries and veins which branch out from the disc and supply the transmitting system of retinal cells and fibres, and secondly the choroidal system, which supplies the receptors, the rods and cones.

One would expect this double blood-supply would give the retina extra protection but this is not the case. If *either* system fails the situation is bad and in many cases disastrous. This is because the individual retinal arteries do not anastomose (link-up) with neighbouring vessels. The blood-supply to any organ of the body has three components: the blood-vessels, the blood cells, and the plasma, the fluid in which they float. A lesion (fault) in any one of the three has profound effects on the other two.

Diseases of retinal blood-vessels

Diabetic retinopathy is an excellent example of the relationship of these three factors. There are the changes in the larger vessels leading to the formation of new vessels, damaged capillaries leak blood and plasma into the retinal tissues, and the lipoids (fats) in the plasma are deposited in the retinal layers as hard exudates. (This condition is described fully on p. 16).

Arteriosclerosis (loss of elasticity) of the retinal vessels usually occurs in middle life and later. It may be associated with raised blood-pressure (hypertension) or kidney disease. Arteriosclerosis is usually accompanied by a deposition of material in the inner walls of the arterioles. The effect on the blood-flow is similar to that of a water supply when the pipes fur up — a slowing up or a complete blockage.

Venous thrombosis, or thrombosis of the central retinal vein, comes on suddenly and the only symptom noticed by the patient is a loss of vision. There is never any pain. The diagnosis is made easily by examination of the fundus (Fig. 2). The veins are much wider than usual and the disc is swollen. There are hundreds of small retinal haemorrhages scattered over the entire fundus. Sometimes only one of the four veins is obstructed (branch thrombosis) and in these cases the haemorrhages are confined to one sector. The outlook for vision is very poor. A complication may also have to be faced about three months after the thrombosis: secondary glaucoma (p. 52). This is caused by new vessels on the surface of the iris and in the angle of the anterior chamber, blocking the outflow of intra-ocular fluid.

Occlusion of the central retinal artery is often caused by arteriosclerosis but there are two other conditions which give a similar clinical picture: temporal arteritis and embolus. In all cases the onset is sudden and the only symptom loss of vision. The fundus picture shows extreme narrowing of the retinal vessels and sometimes clumps of blood cells can be seen moving in a jerky manner (cattle-trucking). This is never seen under normal conditions. The posterior pole is milky white, a response to lack of oxygen, and the macula shows up in the middle of it as a 'cherry-spot'. Recovery is unlikely but secondary glaucoma is rare.

Temporal arteritis Temporal (giant-cell) arteritis is usually found in older people. It is an inflammatory disease of the walls of blood-vessels in many parts of the body and it gets its name because it frequently selects the temporal arteries, which run a tortuous course over the temples of the head. The ophthalmic arteries, which provide the main vascular supply to the eyes, may also be involved and through them the central retinal arteries.

The disease usually comes to notice through an occlusion of the central retinal artery of one or other side; the symptoms and signs are exactly the same as any other central artery occlusion. What *is* different however is that the second eye is very liable to develop the same condition so that complete blindness may result. The condition must always be suspected when arterial occlusion occurs in an elderly person and the diagnosis is helped by finding tenderness on the side of the head and by the laboratory test, the blood sedimentation rate, which is much raised in temporal arteritis. Sometimes the diagnosis has to be established by

25

the removal of a small part of the temporal artery which is examined
for the presence of giant cells with the microscope (biopsy). If the disease is present the patient must start taking oral steroids to prevent the
second eye becoming blind.

Embolus of the central retinal artery or one of its main branches
again gives a very similar picture to other arterial occlusions of the central retinal artery. An embolus is a small fragment of the tissue lining
the wall of one of the larger arteries (the carotid usually in the case of
the eye) which has broken away and has been carried along the arterial
system into smaller and smaller blood-vessels as the artery branches.
Finally it gets to a branch a little narrower than itself and there it sticks.
Sometimes this happens in the main trunk of the central retinal artery
just behind the optic disc and sometimes, if it is even smaller and lodges
in the retina itself, it shows as a tiny white mass at the point where the
artery divides. It is occasionally possible to persuade the embolus to
pass on to an even smaller vessel where it does less harm. The best way
to do this is to massage the eyeball with the finger tip for several minutes through the closed upper lid using moderately firm pressure.

There are two other conditions which are caused by inflammatory
changes in the walls of the retinal blood-vessels. These are Eale's disease
(Dr Eale was a Birmingham physician) and Behcet's disease (Professor
Behcet was a Turkish dermatologist).

Eale's disease (perivasculitis) is found mainly in men aged from 20 to
30. Cases are most common in the Middle East. Both eyes are usually
affected. The periphery of the fundi is the favourite place for the lesions.
The small blood-vessels here begin to bleed and connective tissue forms
around their walls. This drags the vessels out of position and causes
more bleeding and often new-vessel formation. In time the disease
'burns itself out' but often not before there has been considerable
damage to the retina. Photocoagulation (see p. 15) is often helpful in
Eale's disease as the trouble spots can be eradicated completely. Unfortunately fresh areas of activity keep breaking out. The cause of
Eale's disease is unknown.

Behcet's disease is also prevalent in the Middle East and, again, the
cause is unknown but men are more frequently affected than women.
The patient suffers from recurrent attacks of diminished vision associated with widespread blockage of the smaller retinal vessels. It is often

associated with recurrent uveitis with hypopyon and ulceration of the mouth and genitalia. Both eyes are usually involved and the condition often progresses to blindness. Treatment in the active stages is by oral steroids. If uveitis is present it is treated on the lines described in p. 46 and hypopyon as on p. 34.

Diseases of blood cells

Diseases of the blood cells, such as pernicious anaemia and leukaemia, often give rise to retinal haemorrhages. This is because they have a harmful effect on the endothelial cells lining the capillary blood-vessels. These conditions do not often cause impaired vision unless a haemorrhage occurs right at the macula.

Sickle-cell haemoglobin C disease, on the other hand, is a not-infrequent cause of loss of vision. The disease is confined to Negroes, particularly those living in East Africa. But, like onchocerciasis, p. 102, it was carried by the slave trade across the Atlantic to Central America and the West Indies.

Sickle-cell disease is caused by an abnormality in the haemoglobin of the red blood cells which makes the cells take on an elongated sickle-shaped form. They are also stiffer than normal so that they cannot squeeze through the capillary vessels as they should. This causes blockage (capillary thromboses). The blockages take place in those parts where the blood-flow is normally slow, and the small blood-vessels at the periphery of the retinae are liable to be affected.

The lesions are similar to those found in Eale's disease. There are small retinal haemorrhages, connective tissue, and, later, new-vessel formations. A vitreous haemorrhage from one of these calls attention to the disease. The haemorrhages are often massive and recurrent, involving both eyes. Cold, low oxygen pressure (e.g. in aeroplanes), and alcoholic intoxication are all liable to bring on a fresh series of capillary thromboses and special precautions are taken should an anaesthetic have to be administered. Photocoagulation is of limited help in eradicating the sites of new vessel formations. One eye is often more seriously involved than the other and blindness often results.

Diseases of the plasma

One disease may affect the vision: macroblobulinaemia. In this disease abnormal proteins in the plasma cause it to become very viscid. This slows blood-flow and results in a lack of oxygen in all parts of the body. Both fundi show the same changes; a great distension of the retinal veins with scattered haemorrhages all over the surfaces of the retinae.

Blindness caused by poisons and drugs

Several toxic (poisonous) substances and drugs are responsible for blindness. In most cases something in the individual's make-up causes them to be abnormally sensitive (allergic) to that particular substance. The blindness affects both eyes and in most cases the damage is done to the retina or optic nerve.

Tobacco

Tobacco amblyopia (blindness) is a not-uncommon cause of poor central vision in the over-sixties. Tobacco is a strong and harmful drug. Its addicts are numbered in millions and the number is increasing, especially in the Third World countries where the populations are subjected to subtle and uncontrolled advertising by the tobacco companies.

Tobacco can kill slowly by lung cancer or more speedily by coronary thrombosis: in these conditions the killer is the cigarette. In tobacco amblyopia it is the pipe. The smoker uses strong tobacco and very often takes more alcohol than he should. He is often retired, rather bored with life, and a little bit careless about his appearance. The older text-books referred to him as a 'seedy old gentleman', for the condition is very rare in women.

Tobacco causes a poisoning of the ganglion cells of the retina (Plate 1). The blindness comes on slowly and is never complete, as it is the cells of the macula area which suffer most. The patient notices that reading is becoming difficult and may complain that his wife is looking rather pale or that the house needs painting. The periphery of the retina is unaffected so he has no difficulty in getting about.

As far as the oculist is concerned there is little abnormal to be found when the case is examined in the early stages, and the deterioration of vision is regarded as being due to senile macular degeneration, which it often resembles. Later, however, the disc becomes pale and testing the central visual field for colour reveals a dense scotoma (see p. 17), most marked for a red object.

Disorders of the retina

Treatment is quite effective in restoring sight. The lack of vitamin B_{12} (hydroxocobalamin) is supplied by injections which have to be continued for at least a year; it takes some six months before an improvement is noticeable. The patient should stop smoking.

Methyl alcohol. Methyl alcohol, methylated spirits, and wood alcohol are the cheapest and most effective way of getting blind drunk.

When the victim recovers consciousness he suffers from severe nausea, giddiness, and mental confusion. There may also be any degree of loss of vision. The condition is often mistaken for a severe 'hang-over' but the impaired vision should suggest something more serious.

Methyl alcohol poisoning is much less common than it was 50 years ago. This is mainly due to regulations which prohibit the sale of methylated spirits unless it is adulterated by foul-tasting substances. Even so, desperate alcoholics are able to drink it. It is unfortunately possible to obtain pure methyl alcohol from many sorts of laboratory and a common way in which poisoning occurs is by 'lacing' drinks at a party.

Urgent hospitalization is necessary, for the treatment requires careful and repeated estimations of the blood chemistry together with intravenous infusions.

Iatrogenic blindness. The term 'iatrogenic' is a polite way of saying that doctors have caused a condition, for example when drugs used to combat disease in some other part of the body have an adverse effect on the eyes. Sometimes doctors know the risks they are running; indeed in the case of steroid preparations, given for long-term treatment in conditions such as asthma and arthritis, which may cause cataract, this risk is accepted (p. 40). At other times, when the physician has been alerted to possible side-effects, he keeps a special watch for them and may find it necessary to stop the drug entirely or substitute another. At other times again, and these cases cause considerable concern, the patient has an unusual hypersensitivity (allergy) to the drug. Two drugs in particular which are in current use in general medicine require to be carefully monitored by the oculist. These are chloroquine and ethambutol.

Chloroquine is a synthetic derivative of quinine which itself occasionally causes acute loss of vision in susceptible people. The effect on the eyes of chloroquine, which is used in the treatment of chronic conditions such as rheumatoid arthritis and systemic lupus erythema-

29

tosus occurs only after prolonged treatment of a year or two and reduces central vision in both eyes. There is a very typical fundus appearance, the so-called 'bull's eye' macula caused by degeneration of the pigment cells of that area. Later there is narrowing of the retinal vessels and optic atrophy. Once these appearances are present the vision has been permanently impaired even if the chloroquine is stopped. It is important regularly to examine the fundi and central fields for the first signs of the condition.

Ethambutol is a drug used in tuberculosis, especially in those cases where the bacillus is resistant to the more commonly used drugs such as isoniazid and streptomycin. It can cause inflammation of the optic nerves (optic neuritis) and this causes a central scotoma (see p. 17). The central fields need to be checked regularly if this drug is in use.

4

Disorders of the cornea, aqueous, and vitreous

Rays of light from objects we can see have to pass through the eye to reach the rods and cones of the retina (p. 13). In order to form a clear image on the retina the parts of the eye which transmit the light must be perfectly clear. These structures, or transparent media as they are called, are, from front to back: the cornea, the aqueous, the crystalline lens, and the vitreous gel (or jelly) (Fig. 1).

Structure and function of the cornea

Four hundred million years ago an outstanding evolutionary advance occurred: the cornea developed in fish. This provided a porthole for the brain to view the world: one so effective that Nature to this day has not improved on it.

The cornea is tough and strong and, with the sclera, forms the outer protective coat of the eye. Further its convexity is the basis of the main mechanism by which distant objects are focused on the retina. Above all the cornea is of crystal clarity and transmits light without distortion or scattering.

The cornea, less than 1 millimetre in thickness, is a relatively simple structure and consists of five layers. These layers are shown in the photograph of a cross-section of the cornea (Plate 2). It will be seen that the main bulk of the cornea is the substantia propria. This consists of an immense number of fine but strong fibrils very similar to those found in tendon. In the cornea the fibrils run in the form of bundles of parallel fibres, rather like basket-work; it is the absolute regularity of the arrangement which makes the cornea transparent. Surrounding the fibrils there is a softer transparent material called the ground substance, a sort of 'filling-in' matter.

The front layer of the cornea, the corneal epithelium, is a continuation of the conjunctiva and consists of some six layers of flattened cells. These are loosely attached to Bowman's membrane, a thin transparent

31

layer separating the epithelium from the substantia propria. The back layer of the cornea is a single layer of cells called the endothelium. Despite its frail structure the endothelium is of great importance to the proper functioning of the cornea. Between the endothelium and the substantia propria is an elastic layer called Decemet's membrane.

The hazy cornea

Van Leeuwenhoek (1632–1723) (p. 8) was the first to show that if the cornea was cut away from the rest of the eye and soaked in water two important changes occurred: it swelled to two or three times its original thickness and it became opaque like the eye of a dead fish. Both these appearances are due to the same thing: the cornea has soaked up water. But in the living eye, although the cornea is lying between two films of watery fluid, the tears in front and the aqueous behind, it neither swells nor loses its transparency. Why not? The answer is that in the healthy cornea fluid is continuously being sucked away so that it is dehydrated, or, in other words depleted of water, and this is why it keeps its clarity.

We shall presently see that this dehydration depends largely on having a healthy epithelium in front and a healthy endothelial membrane behind and if there is any injury or disease of either layer the substantia propria immediately starts to draw in water and becomes opaque. Either a generalized haze or discrete areas of corneal opacity are found in many disease states; these cause an obstruction to the passage of the rays of light. When this happens the image of the outside world becomes indistinct in the way that it does from inside a car when a windscreen becomes misted up or dirty.

A uniform haziness of the cornea takes place in a number of pathological conditions. For example the oedema (fluid retention) of the epithelium and substantia propria in conditions of raised intra-ocular pressure (p. 57), the oedema of the endothelium Decemet's membrane and substantia propria which may accompany uveitis (p. 46), or the degenerative conditions of the corneal endothelium and epithelium (corneal dystrophies) which are found mainly in the older age groups.

Localized opacities of the cornea are also found in disease conditions and the most common of these are opacities in the cornea caused by ulcers, inflammations of the substantia propria (deep keratitis), and certain degenerations such as conical cornea or band-shaped opacity of the cornea.

Corneal abrasions and ulcers

The delicate corneal epithelium can easily be stripped away from Bowman's membrane by quite a trivial accident such as a brush from a twig. This causes severe pain and watering. The extent of the abrasion is found by 'staining'. A green dye called fluorescein impregnated on filter paper and placed for a few seconds behind the lower lid will stain the tears and show up the abraded area as a vivid green patch. It heals by multiplication of the epithelial cells at its edge and this usually takes one or two days. It is important to pad the eye, as this promotes healing, and also to instil antibiotic ointment to combat infection (see below).

A recurrent abrasion is not uncommon. After an interval of some weeks, if the epithelium has not adhered firmly to Bowman's membrane during healing, it breaks down again and has to be treated as before. Further recurrences can usually be prevented by instilling ointment every night for six months.

Corneal ulcers usually start as infected abrasions but the break in the epithelium may be so small that it is unnoticed by the patient. However small the break bacteria can gain entry and set up an inflammation. The extent of the ulcerated area is found by 'staining' as has been described for corneal abrasions. Surrounding the ulcer is a greyish halo caused by excess fluid in the epithelium and substantia propria; once again, the cornea loses its transparency when it takes up too much water. The blood-vessels surrounding the cornea become engorged and some even penetrate its substance to help in the healing process.

The treatment is to combat any infection present by means of antibiotics (such as chloramphenicol or gentamicin) and to put the muscles inside the eye at rest by using atropine drops. The eye is padded until it no longer stains. Rapid healing of the ulcer is all important. If the ulcer passes the barrier of Bowman's membrane a permanent scar is formed. This is because the fibrils of the substantia propria are damaged and lose their regular arrangement. If the scar involves the central part of the cornea a greater or lesser degree of sight is certain to be lost but clarity can be restored by grafting a circular disc from a cadaver eye (keratoplasty).

There are two types of corneal ulcer which deserve special mention. These are the hypopyon and dendritic ulcers. The hypopyon ulcer is a large, destructive ulcer of a yellowish colour caused by particularly virulent strains of bacteria. These cause an inflammation of the structures inside the eye, particularly the iris, with the result that white blood cells (which protect the body against bacterial invaders) pour into the anterior chamber and sink to the bottom, forming a yellow–grey deposit with a horizontal fluid level, the hypopyon. This indicates a very severe infection and besides the measures already described needs antibiotics (gentamicin 20 mg, repeated daily) injected under the conjunctiva. In this way a high concentration inside the eye is obtained. Before the discovery of antibiotics the presence of a hypopyon always indicated that that eye would soon have to be removed but now this is rarely necessary and in fact most of them recover with useful vision. (see p. 62).

Dendritic ulcers are quite another matter, and are transmitted by contact (for example, when a mother kisses her baby) with someone with a 'cold-sore'. A 'cold-sore' indicates that a person has a virus called herpes simplex living in the skin. Under normal conditions it lies dormant, but a running nose, a little sunburn, or a scratch sets up a vesicle (pus pimple) on the skin around the mouth or nose, usually a scab forms and no treatment is necessary, but sometimes the virus gets into the cornea and from time to time breaks out into an ulcer with an easily recognizable form: the dendritic ulcer, because of its resemblance to the branching of a tree. It is slow to heal, very apt to be recurrent, and can form fine scars anywhere on the cornea. Sometimes a uveitis (p. 45) is also set up.

These ulcers are treated on the usual lines except that there are certain drugs (idoxuridine) which act directly on the virus. But, of course prevention is better than cure. It is quite likely that infected mothers of today got *their* herpes simplex infection from the cold sores of their own mothers.

Other corneal opacities

Other conditions cause localized corneal opacities and loss of vision. Congenital syphilis is often associated with a severe inflammation of the substantia propria of both eyes. The condition usually comes on acutely at the age of from 5 to 10 years. There is extreme pain and watering in the acute stage, which lasts several months. The eyes become blind as the oedema, which causes a greyish opacity, gradually involves the whole cornea. Then there is a stage when new blood-vessels grow into the cornea from the periphery following which the opacity slowly clears, leaving a diffuse scarring of the corneae and greatly reduced vision. In the acute stages steroid drops and atropine are the most effective treatment. Years later when all inflammation has died out vision may be restored by corneal grafting. Other forms of this so-called deep keratitis are caused by tuberculosis and herpes simplex. These usually affect one eye only.

Band-shaped opacity is a degenerative condition. As its name suggests it takes the form of a band across the cornea. The epithelium and front part of the substantia propria are involved. In the developed countries the condition is usually associated with a chronic uveitis but a similar condition is also found in people who have had excessive exposure to ultraviolet light; the Eskimos suffer the condition because of light reflected from snow, and pearl divers in the Pacific from the reflection from water and white sand. The condition can be treated surgically.

Many other localized corneal lesions reduce the sight but they are relatively uncommon and rarely cause blindness. They include scars following wounds of the cornea, and degenerative conditions (dystrophies) which may occur in any of the five layers. If the opacity is the result of scarring any sight which may have been lost can be restored by corneal grafting. In the operation of corneal grafting a disc of the diseased opaque cornea is removed by a trephine (an instrument with the same principle as an apple-corer, with a cutting edge on the lower end of a hollow cylinder) and replaced by a similar disc from a cadaver eye. The disc is either the full thickness of the cornea (penetrating graft) or just the front layers (lamellar graft) and varies in size from 6 to 9 mm in diameter. The donor graft is sutured in place by very fine nylon thread.

The aqueous

The aqueous is the space between the back surface of the cornea and the front surface of the lens. It is divided by the iris into the anterior and posterior chamber and is filled with intra-ocular fluid. Its formation and function is described on p. 50.

Normally the aqueous is perfectly clear but after injury or surgery it may be full of red blood cells (hyphaema, p. 63) or, in cases of hypopyon, of white blood cells (p. 34). In cases of uveitis these cells can often be seen by the slit-lamp (p. 46).

The vitreous

The vitreous is a transparent gel (or jelly) which occupies the interior of the globe behind the lens. In young people it fills the space completely and is firmly adherent to the optic disc behind and to the region of the suspensory ligament in front. Elsewhere it is attached to the retina by fine fibrils. A decade or so ago the vitreous was regarded as a simple, rather firm, jelly filling an empty space and acting as a support to the retina; but electron microscope studies have shown it to have a complex structure consisting of very fine fibrils embedded in a softer transparent material. It also contains cells, especially in those parts adjacent to the retina. These cells have the ability to change their form and also their function. Sometimes they act as 'scavenger' cells, disposing of unwanted matter such as bacteria or dead tissue. In certain disease conditions these vitreous cells take part in the formation of bands of connective tissue in the interval between the vitreous and retina.

The vitreous may lose its clarity either because of changes in its structure which occur in degenerative conditions, or because particles of opaque matter invade its substance.

The vitreous often starts to degenerate when people reach middle life and the most common change of this nature is the formation of fluid spaces in the firm gel (fluid vitreous). This condition is benign but it may cause surgical difficulties should a cataract operation be required later. Another degenerative change is called retraction of the vitreous. In this condition the vitreous shrinks away from the retina so that there is a space between them filled by intra-ocular fluid. The retraction may involve a small area, usually in the region of the posterior pole, or be very extensive, involving the whole vitreous. These eyes usually see perfectly well but once the firm support of the vitreous gel is lost there is an increased liability to retinal detachment.

Disorders of the cornea, aqueous, and vitreous

Vitreous degeneration is also common in the higher degrees of myopia when the elongation of the fibrous coats draws the retina away from the vitreous.

Vitreous floaters

In all these degenerations the vitreous fibrils tend to coalesce into particles of denser matter suspended in the gel. These are commonly known as 'floaters'. They may be of any size up to that of the diameter of the optic disc and are frequently multiple. They can often be seen by the patient as semi-transparent objects which move in a swinging motion when the eye moves. They are best seen silhouetted against a light background such as a grey sky. Sometimes the 'floater' is very well defined with a recognizable form like a string of bubbles or a tadpole (muscae volitantes).

Some vitreous floaters are visible for months or even years, but eventually they float away into oblivion. They can be seen quite easily with an ophthalmoscope. Although 'floaters' rarely interfere with vision their presence always implies the need for a careful check-up on the retina as sometimes a retinal hole or early detachment can give rise to very similar symptoms.

Blood cells in the vitreous

Bleeding into the vitreous occurs only in pathological conditions such as diabetic retinopathy, Eale's disease (p. 26), sickle-cell disease (p. 27), and contusion of the eyeball (p. 63). Sometimes the blood forms a pocket between the retina and back surface of the vitreous (sub-hyaloid haemorrhage) and sometimes it breaks through into the vitreous jelly. The effect on vision depends on the quantity of the blood and whether it lies in the central area or nearer the periphery. Sometimes the bleeding takes many months to clear; in some instances up to two years with recovery of vision. This has given rise to the ophthalmologists' adage: 'never despair of a vitreous haemorrhage'.

Vitreous haemorrhages, however, are apt to form dense membranes in the vitreous and retina and these with the secondary cataracts which also form, may ruin vision even if the haemorrhage clears. If the haemorrhage persists for over a year it is usual to remove it together with the retained clot (vitrectomy operation).

White blood cells are frequently found in the vitreous in cyclitis and choroiditis p. 47, in which they form a cloud of minute opacities; later these coalesce into denser floaters. The treatment of these is that of the underlying uveitis.

5

Disorders of the crystalline lens

Structure and function of the crystalline lens

The crystalline lens has a small central core which is formed in the early weeks of the life of the embryo; as growth proceeds further tissue is laid down to surround it like the layers of an onion. Its growth goes on throughout life. This means that the first-formed (or oldest) lens tissue lies buried in the centre and the more recently formed tissue is near the surface of the lens. The lens tissue consists of long transparent fibrils which interlock before and behind. Surrounding the lens is its capsule. This is an elastic covering to which is attached the suspensory ligament of the lens. This ligament is seen in Fig. 3 (p. 51) and runs from the equator of the lens to the ciliary processes.

The main function of the lens is to provide a variable focusing device which enables images of objects at differing distance from the eye to be accurately aligned on the retina. When the ring of ciliary processes contracts, the suspensory ligament slackens and the lens, which is elastic, becomes more convex; this brings the image of nearer objects to a focus on the retina. Conversely, when the ring slackens, the ligament becomes more taut and the lens curvatures become less convex so that distant objects can now come to a focus on the retina. This variation in the focus goes on unceasingly throughout the waking hours.

Cataracts

When the lens becomes opaque it is said to have a cataract. It must be clearly understood that a cataract is *any* opacity in the lens, large or small, and it may form at any time in the life of the individual from embryonic life to old age.

A cataract occurs because there is some disturbance to the nutrition of the lens; most commonly a lack of oxygen. The lens has no blood-vessels of its own and has to rely on the oxygen and other nutrients brought to it in the intra-ocular fluid. In the elderly, particularly, there is a shortage of oxygen in the intra-ocular fluid because the blood-vessels of retina and choroid gradually constrict with age.

The most common form of cataract therefore is that found in old age; the so-called 'senile' cataract. This kind of cataract can hardly be classified as a disease, indeed it is no more so than the hair turning white. The term 'senile' is unfortunate as the word has a connotation with mental deterioration which of course these people in no way have. But there are many other types of cataract.

Congenital cataracts are present at birth. They are often associated with other eye defects (see p. 90), and may run in families. Others are due to interference to the growth of the developing lens, which can be caused by all sorts of harmful influences, for example rubella cataract. This cataract is formed in the early weeks of embryonic life (particularly between the sixth and twelfth weeks after conception) if the mother is infected by the rubella (German measles) virus. Both eyes of the developing fetus develop cataracts and often the retinae are damaged as well. Other parts of the body may also suffer, the most serious effects being those on the heart and intestinal organs. Often these conditions are not compatible with life and spontaneous abortion takes place. If it does survive the child is not completely blind. The cataracts occupy the very centre of the lens and are often quite small; these are the lens fibres which were attacked by the rubella virus. The next fibres to be laid down are transparant because they have not been so affected. The central cataracts remain unchanged throughout life, 'like flies in amber'. Like other congenital cataracts they may need surgery but the visual results are often disappointing because of the retinal damage caused by the virus.

If a woman has not had German measles before child-bearing age contact with a case during the early months of pregnancy should be avoided at all cost. Traumatic cataract, caused by injury to the lens, is described on p. 61.

Endocrine cataracts can occur, and are some ten times more common in diabetics than in the population at large. Another form of endocrine cataract sometimes follows the prolonged treatment with steroids necessary in certain chronic conditions such as asthma and rheumatoid arthritis (see also lamellar cataract and cataract in galactocaemia, cretinism and Mongols' pp. 90 and 91).

Symptoms

The symptoms of cataract are entirely visual and the most common is that there is a lack of definition; patients often say 'newsprint is very indistinct nowadays', or they find that colours become very dull and say: 'the house needs painting'. There is also a difference in the colours that are seen by cataractous eyes; if you look at a Rembrandt painting done in his old age you will find a preponderance of browns and reds; contrast it with a painting by Van Gogh, who died aged 47, and whose paintings are splashings of blues, greens, and yellows, the colours of shorter wavelengths. Cataract plays other tricks on the sight. The eyes sometimes become short-sighted so that although distant objects may be out of focus the patient begins to see near objects more distinctly again. But unfortunately this happy state of affairs does not last for ever and even near sight becomes obscured. Again, double vision sometimes occurs when a cataract splits the entering beam of light. Finally, dazzle in bright light is a common symptom caused in much the same way as dust on a windscreen.

If the cause of poor vision in an older person is found to be cataract they must be told because the outlook in cataract cases is good. The rate at which the cataract forms is very variable and they often 'stop in their tracks' for years. As a general rule the later in life a cataract appears the slower is its progress. A cataract is not removed immediately it causes visual loss as other factors have to be taken into account such as the degree of cataract and loss of vision in the other eye. It may well be that in the aged person with a limited environment, who can see enough to enjoy television (which can usually be seen long after reading becomes impossible), operation will never be required at all. Sometimes, however, a cataract has to be removed because it becomes hypermature (over-ripe) and causes inflammation. This type of lens change shows as a whitish opacity in the pupil and is often seen in dogs. Incidentally these dense white cataracts give the condition its name. Just as a cascade of water rushing through a narrow gorge becomes white with foam so the normally transparent 'waters of the eye', as the ancients called the lens and vitreous humours, become opaque.

Treatment

Despite numerous claims by quack practitioners, the treatment of cataract is surgical. The success rate is high: about 97 per cent of operations give greatly improved vision, but as in any other surgical operation it is never possible to guarantee a perfect result. The surgeons who claim their patients have no complications are those who do not do much surgery!

The aim of the operation is either to remove the crystalline lens entirely (total removal) or to leave the outer layer of the capsule and remove the remaining 98 per cent of lens tissue inside it (subtotal removal). Both methods have their indications.

Most cataract operations are carried out under general anaesthesia; this is usually preferred both by surgeon and patient as any involuntary movement on the part of the latter is not possible. However, if there are any medical contra-indications the operation can be carried out painlessly under a local anaesthetic.

At operation an incision is made extending nearly half way round the periphery of the cornea, and the cataractous lens is gently drawn out through the dilated pupil. After this the incision is closed by fine silk or nylon thread which is often left in for life.

Patients are usually out of bed the day following operation but are not allowed to bend their heads or do any form of lifting as this may cause the complication of haemorrhage. There are promising new techniques, at present available at only a few centres, in which the lens is broken up and sucked out of a very small incision (phaecoemulsification). This further reduces the time spent in hospital; indeed there are some centres where the operation is an out-patient procedure.

Cataract in children and young adults is treated by a less elaborate technique in which the lens capsule is opened by a fine needle and allowing the intra-ocular fluid to soften the lens material which is subsequently sucked away.

After removal of cataract the eye is said to be 'aphakic' and optically speaking becomes very long-sighted. With a suitable high-powered 'plus' lens the patient sees well again and temporary 'plus' lenses can often be ordered while the patient is still in hospital. The refraction of the eye, however, alters steadily in the first few months after operation and it is 3–4 months before permanent glasses for distance and another pair for near work can be ordered. There may be further problems: the alteration in refraction makes objects appear to be much nearer than they really are and much too large. Sometimes vertical lines like doorways appear to be curved. And the patient may have had for years an indistinct image of their own face in the mirror or that of their spouses and after their operation the odd wrinkle or the few odd lip hairs are clearly seen, perhaps all too clearly!

Although conventional glasses give a somewhat distorted image in some people, most get adjusted as the months go by. There are however two ways in which normal images can be obtained. The first is by wearing a contact lens, and 'continuous-wear' contact lenses are now available, or, at the time of the original operation, a tiny plastic lens (ocular insert) can be put into the eye. This can be extremely effective but does introduce an added risk, albeit a small one, to the operation.

For mass cataract operations in developing countries see p. 99.

6

Disorders of the uveal tract

Uveitis

The term uveitis means an inflammation of the uveal tract. The cross
section of the eyeball (Fig. 1) shows the uveal tract lying between
the sclera and retina and, as it is largely composed of blood-vessels, it is
called the vascular coat of the eye. The uveal tract consists of three
structures closely linked by their intertwining blood-vessels. The front
part of the tract is the iris, the function of which is to vary the size of
the pupil. The middle part is the ciliary body, with two main functions:
first it is responsible for the formation of the intra-ocular fluid, and
secondly it controls the accommodation (focusing) of the crystalline
lens. The third and hindermost part is the choroid. Its rôle is to provide
the main blood-supply to the structures inside the eye, especially to the
retina which it surrounds like a mantle. Inflammation of the individual
parts of the uveal tract are known as iritis, cyclitis (if the ciliary body is
involved), and choroiditis. The same disease frequently affects any of
the three parts. Both eyes are often attacked but often not at the same
time. The attacks vary in severity and there is a strong tendency for
them to be recurrent; each episode causing further damage to the eye.
Uveitis is a major cause of blindness in the under-50s.

Causes

Uveitis is a reaction in the eye from some condition outside it. So what
are the possible causes of such a reaction? A mere catalogue of them
would easily fill this page. Furthermore theories about the cause of
uveitis change in every decade. So an oculist writing in 1930 gave a
completely different list from the one I would give in 1982 and doubtless one writing in the year 2000 will smile at our simple beliefs! However, there are some well-proven associations between infections of the
eye by micro-organisms which affect the body as a whole. One of the
most common causes of uveitis is an infection by a microscopic parasite

called *Toxoplasma gondii*. It lies dormant in tissues, especially the uveal tract, for years, erupts into activity to give a fresh attack of uveitis, and then reverts again to its dormant state. Most micro-organisms favour one particular animal host but the toxoplasma is catholic in its taste and causes disease in a variety of creatures including mice and whales. Blood tests show that many of us have at some time been infected by *Toxoplasma*. In most of us this has caused no trouble. Our built-in defences have overcome the infection as they deal with many others — both known and unknown to us.

Taking a global view, two very common causes of uveitis are leprosy and onchocerciasis, the former due to a bacterium and the latter to a filiria, another type of parastic invader. In both cases any or all of the parts of the uveal tract may be involved and in both blindness frequently occurs. These conditions are described more fully in the chapter on blindness in the Third World.

Uveitis is also caused by two of the common venereal diseases, syphilis and gonorrhoea. Blindness from these causes is much less common than it was 40 years ago but as both infections have recently been on the increase again, we can expect to see a rise in incidence and congenital syphilis (passed on by an infected mother during pregnancy) will again take its toll among the young.

Owing to the fact that a remission of uveitis sometimes follows the successful treatment of dental infections, nasal sinusitis, infected tonsils, and other conditions of so-called 'focal sepsis', these places are carefully examined for evidence of active disease but we now think that their importance as causes of uveitis rather overrated and the fashion for wholesale removal of teeth and tonsils has been changed towards more conservative treatment.

Uveitis can be caused by viruses. The association is usually quite obvious. Herpes simplex virus (which causes cold-sores; p. 34) first forms a dendritic ulcer on the cornea and this spreads into the iris and ciliary body. Herpes zoster (shingles) may also give a severe iridocyclitis if it attacks the trigeminal nerve.

Tuberculosis, or consumption, so familiar to the Victorians as a cause of death in young adults is rapidly being stamped out in the Northern hemisphere but much more slowly in the Southern. In the past it was often incriminated as a cause of uveitis but again views have changed. It has a close but not so murderous cousin called sarcoidosis, which is non-infectious. Sarcoidosis attacks particularly the lungs and lymph glands and is quite commonly associated with uveitis involving all or any of the three parts of the uveal tract. Like the lesions elsewhere in the body the uveitis runs a protracted course.

Uveitis is sometimes associated with arthritis (joint inflammation). A particularly severe form occurs in Still's disease, which is found in children. Another association is with rheumatoid arthritis and, much less commonly with a spinal disease called ankylosing spondylitis, and Reiter's disease. These conditions are similar in that their victims are of certain hereditary 'tissue-types' (see also Behcet's disease p. 26).

In over half of the cases of uveitis it is not possible to determine the cause. Sympathetic ophthalmia (p. 000) may provide the clue. Could the uveitis be some sort of allergy? — Moreover an allergy that the patient has developed to his own tissues (a so-called auto-immune reaction)? One pointer which may be of importance is that uveitis of all types respond well to corticosteroids (cortisone and prednisolone) and this is a feature of other conditions in which there is a proven auto-immune basis.

Diagnosis and treatment

The symptoms of uveitis depend largely on which part of the uveal tract is principally involved. If the iris is inflamed the eye is acutely painful and the vision is misty. The eye is red and the iris is discoloured because the blood-vessels are dilated. The pupil is constricted. With the slit-lamp microscope the effects of the iritis can be seen even more clearly. The inflammation causes cells to be passed into the anterior chamber (p. 36) where they can actually be seen as shining particles in the aqueous. It is probable that, in places, the pupil is stuck to the front surface of the crystalline lens against which it rests. This is a dangerous sign: if the adhesions between the pupil margin and the lens become complete the circulation of the intra-ocular fluid will become obstructed at that point and a secondary glaucoma may develop.

If the ciliary body is inflamed (cyclitis) the symptoms are not nearly

46

so dramatic. The vision becomes misty due to inflammatory cells passing into the anterior chamber and the front part of the vitreous humour but the eye is quiet.

In choroiditis the eye again looks normal externally but when the fundus is examined with the ophthalmoscope the changes may be striking. The places where the choroid is inflamed show up as whitish/yellow patches and the vitreous humour is hazy. If one of the patches involves the macula, as often happens in toxoplasmosis, the effects on vision are disastrous. When the choroiditis resolves the patches turn into white scars which remain for life and which may in later life be an aid in the diagnosis of congenital syphilis, onchocerciasis, and other conditions.

A later complication of uveal inflammation is the formation of a secondary cataract.

If the cause of the uveitis can be discovered it must of course be treated and there are effective drugs which can alleviate or cure most of the diseases caused by bacteria and parasites. But besides these general measures the inflamed eye needs locally applied treatment. An important drug used in the treatment of uveitis is atropine (belladonna). This has a twofold effect. First it paralyses the muscles inside the eye so that they are put completely at rest and secondly it dilates the pupil and prevents the formation of the adhesions to the lens so that a secondary glaucoma is less liable to develop. Another important group of drugs are the steroids (hydrocortisone and prednisolone), which have an anti-inflammatory action. They can be used in the form of drops, injection under the conjunctiva, or taken by mouth. However, the treatment of uveitis is far from satisfactory and the condition is responsible for some 12 per cent of cases of blindness and partial sight.

Sympathetic ophthalmia

The most dreaded form of uveitis is a disease called sympathetic ophthalmia, a condition in which an injury to one eye may lead to blindness in both. The injury is caused by a sharp object which penetrates the cornea or sclera and allows harmful bacteria to enter the eye. Within a few hours a uveitis is set up and the eye becomes painful, red, and angry. After an interval of about four weeks, but sometimes much longer, the second eye in its turn develops a severe uveitis and, despite

47

treatment, the sight in both may be lost. (see Louis Braille p. 197).

It is believed that the second eye, sometimes called the sympathising eye, becomes allergic to the tissues of the eye which was first inflamed (an auto-immune reaction, see p. 46). The only way to prevent this calamity is to remove the injured eye. If this is done within a fortnight of the accident the risk of involvement of the second eye is very slight, but every day that operation is postponed the risk of sympathetic ophthalmia increases.

Penetrating eye injuries are therefore always a matter of grave concern and their management calls for considerable skill and experience. Much depends on the damage that has been done to the eye at the time of the original injury. For if key structures like the cornea crystalline lens and retina have been wounded the vision is likely always to be poor and the risk involved in keeping the eye is too great. Another important factor that has to be taken into account is the response of the injured eye to treatment. If the eye remains red and irritable and fails to improve with intensive treatment this is a danger sign and calls for its removal.

Against this rather gloomy background it should be said that, thanks to modern surgical techniques, injured eyes recover vision far better than formerly: moreover great advances have been made on the medical side of treatment especially by the use of steroids and other anti-inflammatory drugs. These may save the day when sympathetic ophthalmia has actually occurred. In the Napoleonic wars sympathetic ophthalmia was common, but during the whole of the Middle East campaign in the Second World War not a single case occurred, despite many penetrating injuries. There was however a notable exception. We saw several cases among Sikh soldiers who, for religious reasons, refused to have their injured eyes removed.

Malignant melanoma

The most common cancer of the eyeball is a pigmented tumour of the uveal tract, the malignant melanoma. Usually it occurs in the choroid but it may arise in the iris or ciliary body. These tumours are believed to arise from Schwann cells (found in nerve fibres) and their name melanoma derives from the fact that they contain brown pigment.

Malignant melanoma are most common after the age of 60 and usually occur in one eye only. On the surface of the iris they are seen as dark brown patches. However, there are other marks of similar appearance called naevi or pigmented moles which are very common and are quite innocent. Malignant melanomata increase in size and often distort the pupil margin but moles do not alter in appearance over the years.

In the case of melanoma of the choroid the tumour gradually increases in size and if it lies near the macula it will cause defective vision. It is easily seen with the ophthalmoscope as a dark raised swelling. At other times the retina is detached, and a visual field defect is caused corresponding to the detachment (see p. 21). Tumours of the ciliary body are the least common and are sometimes seen as a black mass in the angle of the anterior chamber.

As melanomata typically only affect one eye there is not a great risk of blindness but there is a danger of spread to other parts like the liver by way of the bloodstream. For this reason it is usually necessary to remove the affected eye. In other cases it is possible to treat the tumour by irradiation of the globe. Iris tumours have the best outlook as they are often seen at an early stage and can be completely removed surgically.

7

Glaucoma

A football needs to be inflated in order to keep its shape. In the same way the eyeball has to maintain an inner pressure in order to keep its rounded form. In the case of the eyeball the pressure is maintained by fluid formed inside the eye, the intra-ocular fluid. The need for a pressure inside the eye is evident when we look at what happens when it falls. If, for example, the eyeball is penetrated by flying glass from a windscreen it immediately loses its pressure and becomes soft. The cornea and sclera then become buckled and when this happens the eye can no longer function as a camera as it is impossible to focus a sharp image on the retina. Everything appears distorted. The pressure inside an eye is called its tension; in this instance we say the tension is low.

In glaucoma, on the other hand the pressure inside the eye is too high; the tension is raised. This is a serious condition and can be caused in many different ways. The first question that we shall discuss is: how is the pressure inside the eyeball kept at the right level under normal conditions?

Formation and circulation of intra-ocular fluid

There is a delicate balance between the amount of fluid (the intra-ocular fluid) formed inside the eye and the amount of fluid which drains away out of the eye. The intra-ocular fluid is manufactured by the ciliary body. It consists almost entirely of water but has some sugar, oxygen, and other substances dissolved in it. The fluid permeates slowly through the structures inside the eyeball, especially those structures such as the lens and vitreous which have no blood-vessels and depend for their nourishment on the oxygen and sugar brought by the intra-ocular fluid. The same fluid also passes between the front of the lens and the back of the iris, through the pupil and into the anterior chamber where it is called the aqueous humour. Here it has a very important function: it nourishes the back surface of the cornea or corneal endothelium. The amount of intra-ocular fluid formed throughout the day is fairly constant.

What of the other side of the balance: the drainage out of the eye? Figure 3 is drawn from a photograph, magnified about 50 times, of the all-important part of the eye which concerns glaucoma: the filtration angle or angle of the anterior chamber. The 'angle' refers to the meeting-point of two structures, the cornea in front and the iris behind. It continues round the anterior chamber. Right at the apex of the angle is an important structure called the trabeculum. This is a narrow band of tissue lying between the anterior chamber and the canal of Schlemm. It is in fact a drain with a filter in it. The filter is made up of a number of fine passages or pores through which the intra-ocular fluid has to pass to get into the canal of Schlemm. From the canal the intra-ocular fluid passes into 'collecting-channels' and from these into the veins lying on the surface of the sclera and from there it escapes into the general circulation. It is the size of the pores in the trabeculum that holds up the flow of intra-ocular fluid sufficiently to maintain the normal intra-

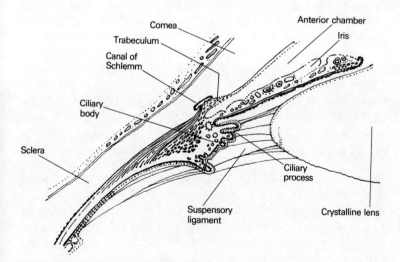

Fig. 3. The angle of the anterior chamber magnified 50 times.

ocular pressure. This is relatively high: usually between 14 and 22 millimetres of mercury (mm Hg). This value varies from person to person and depends on the instrument that is used to measure it.

Even the smallest obstruction to the flow of intra-ocular fluid, anywhere from the ciliary body to its final point of discharge into the surface veins, will cause the pressure to rise above the normal level, making that eye glaucomatous. Sometimes the pressure in the eye becomes raised because of disease of the eye itself. In iritis, for instance, we have already seen how the flow of intra-ocular fluid through the pupil may be obstructed by adhesions between the back surface of the iris and the crystalline lens. Or a tumour growing inside the eye could press the iris against the back of the cornea and obliterate the angle of the anterior chamber. Sometimes after there has been bleeding into the anterior chamber from injury or operation on the iris (hyphaema p. 63) the red cells clog up the pores of the trabeculum so that the intra-ocular fluid cannot escape into the canal of Schlemm. All these are examples of *secondary* glaucoma: they are the result of some other eye disease. One could cite many more examples.

There are also two types of *'primary'* glaucoma; In primary glaucoma the raised pressure is caused by a 'built-in' ocular defect rather than some other eye disease. This defect only gradually becomes apparent, usually towards middle-life. Both eyes are usually affected; one is often more advanced than the other. The two types of primary glaucoma are called open-angle and closed-angle glaucoma respectively. The angle referred to is the angle of the anterior chamber. I shall discuss open-angle glaucoma first; here the angle is exactly the same as it is in the normal eye.

Chronic simple glaucoma

Open-angle glaucoma is often known as wide-angle glaucoma but more commonly still as chronic simple glaucoma. About 1.5 per cent of adults suffer from it and it accounts for some 12 per cent of all registered blind.

In chronic simple glaucoma the tiny pores in the trabeculum get smaller and smaller as the patient ages, and the pressure of the intra-ocular fluid has to rise to compensate for this. It is not a disease in the usually accepted use of the word: it is the body's compensation for the obstruction. It is the most insidious of conditions: over the years the tension gradually rises over the normal 12–24 mm Hg to reach levels in the upper 20s to 30 mm Hg, and often higher.

The effect of long-continued strain is always the same. Something has to give. The effect of prolonged raised pressure on the eye is that the weakest part, in this case the nerve head (optic disc), starts to bulge outwards. This bulging which can be seen with the ophthalmoscope, is called cupping. In the region of the nerve head the nerve fibres from the retina come together in bundles to form the optic nerve. In order to allow these bundles to leave the eye the sclera is perforated in the region of the optic disc. This perforated area is called the lamina cribrosa and is the weakest part of the globe. As the cupping gets more marked another change starts to take place: the capillary blood-vessels are stretched and eventually no longer contain blood. The optic nerve head then becomes white, a change again seen with the ophthalmoscope, and the condition is called optic atrophy. This always causes a marked loss of vision.

The great danger of chronic simple glaucoma is that there are no warning symptoms and quite marked loss of vision is liable to occur before the patient notices anything wrong. Most cases are picked up on routine examinations for glasses, as ophthalmic surgeons and opticians are trained to look out for signs of early cupping. However, some normal people have a similar appearance and some people have glaucoma without cupping, so it is often impossible to be sure that the condition is pathological. Other evidence is therefore needed.

The 'give-away' test for chronic simple glaucoma is the actual measurement of the intra-ocular pressure: tonometry, using instruments called tonometers. There are many types but the principle of all is the same. If you indent a small rubber ball with your thumb you will be able to make a bigger indentation if the ball is soft than if it is hard. Tonometers measure the amount of indentation produced when a known weight or force is applied to the cornea, which is the easiest part of the eye to press on. The intra-ocular pressure can then be calculated, and if it is above 24 mm Hg the eye probably has glaucoma. But one still cannot be absolutely sure. Sometimes the eyeball is abnormally rigid and the reading is a false one. Sometimes a person has a pressure above the normal but even after many years shows no other signs of glaucoma. This condition is known as ocular hypertension and needs no treatment. But it is rare.

Glaucoma cases pass slowly from a high normal pressure to higher and higher pathological pressures and the symptoms usually follow the same pattern. Initially the nerve fibres which arch above the macula are involved and then those below it. This is often unnoticed by the patient as the fibres from the macula itself are not affected. Gradually, however, the defect in the field of vision (the panorama of the world which we see with each eye) (p. 13) extends to the outer parts so the sufferer starts to bump into objects and has difficulty in getting about in the dark. Finally, in untreated cases, the person goes completely blind.

When chronic simple glaucoma has been diagnosed it must be explained to the patient that regular observation is going to be necessary for life. Any visual field loss which has taken place is going to be permanent and the aim of the treatment is to prevent further loss.

As raised pressure in the eye is the root of the trouble the aim of treatment is to reduce that pressure to normal limits. The first line of attack is medical rather than surgical. Very effective eyedrops are available which, if instilled two or three times a day, will lower the intra-ocular pressure. The best-known of them all is pilocarpine used in 1–4 per cent solution. Although it has been in use for over a century its mechanism of action is still unknown. In some way it opens the pores of the trabeculum and allows the intra-ocular fluid to escape from the eye more easily. Pilocarpine has very few side effects and its pressure-lowering effect is strong. However, it does make the pupil very small so patients often find that things look shadowy and that the colours are less dense than before. As less light enters the eye, they may also have difficulties in the dark.

There are alternatives. One type of drop commonly used is 1 per cent adrenalin. Adrenalin also lowers the pressure but not as effectively as pilocarpine. It has the advantage, however, that it does not constrict the pupil. Another new drug is 0.25–0.50 per cent timolol, which lowers tension better than pilocarpine in some cases and does not constrict the pupil. The surgeon finds by trial and error which drops and at which strength most effectively keep the pressure within normal limits, often using them in combination. Certain drugs taken by mouth also lower

54

the ocular pressure. These are called acetazolomides (e.g. Diamox). They are most effective, as we shall see, in acute glaucoma but they have a limited use in chronic simple glaucoma, usually used in combination with eye drops.

In many eyes it is not possible to keep the intra-ocular pressure within normal limits with drops and there is therefore a gradual loss of visual field. It is then necessary to reduce the pressure by operation. Those most commonly performed are the so-called filtering operations. The underlying principle is to create an artificial drainage from the anterior chamber. The drainage is done in the area of the trabeculum, which is bypassed so the intra-ocular fluid passes directly from the anterior chamber to a pocket between the conjunctiva and sclera. The bypass is called a filtering bleb. From the pocket the fluid is absorbed into the neighbouring veins. The originator of the idea was an English surgeon in the Indian Medical Service named Eliot. He made his channel by means of a trephine, a cylindrical tube with a cutting edge at one end which acts like an apple corer. A round disc of tissue 1.5–2.0 millimeters in diameter is removed just where the cornea and sclera meet (often called the limbus). In other operations a tiny trap door is fashioned at the limbus, its closure is prevented by tucking a small piece of iris into the hinge (iris inclusion operation). It is also possible to excise out the trabeculum and let the intra-ocular fluid pass directly into the canal of Schlemm (trabeculectomy).

After a satisfactory filtering operation the pressure is usually well below normal and no further field loss occurs. However, any field which has already been lost is very unlikely to be recovered and the patient and relatives must be forewarned of this.

Narrow-angle glaucoma

The second type of primary glaucoma is the so-called narrow-angle (closed-angle) glaucoma. There is a fundamental difference in the anterior chamber contour in the two types of primary glaucoma. In the narrow-angle type, apart from the fact that the angle between the iris and cornea is narrow, the front of the lens is much closer to the cornea, and the lens is the villain of the piece.

Throughout life the lens gradually grows, putting on fresh layers like an onion. As it grows it pushes the iris farther and farther towards the cornea, making an already narrow angle even narrower, until it is reduced to a narrow chink. Now if the pupil is dilated, as happens in semi-darkness, its front surface can actually touch the back of the cornea, blocking the flow of intra-ocular fluid to the trabeculum. The pressure starts to rise immediately, and the patient is said to be suffering an attack of sub-acute glaucoma. The pressure rises rapidly and can attain values of 50–60 mm Hg. This is a potentially serious situation.

The patient often notices distinctive symptoms. For example the sequence of events might occur something like this:

A middle-aged housewife has an argument with her husband, which makes her very angry. This stimulates the secretion of adrenalin which causes her pupils to dilate. She decides to go by herself to the cinema. The strong emotions engendered by the film, and the darkened condition of the theatre, make her pupils become even more dilated, and the angles of the anterior chamber close. Immediately the intra-ocular pressure starts to rise and by the end of the show has reached a very high level. The eye is not painful but rather uncomfortable and the vision misty. On the walk home, all the street lamps appear to have rings of colour around them, like little rainbows. Similar rainbow rings are apparent around car headlights and other sources of light. The woman is in the throes of an attack of sub-acute glaucoma. If an oculist could see her he would find the cornea to be quite hazy and the pupil dilated. When she gets home, she goes to the kitchen, switches on the light, and makes a cup of tea. Half an hour later the eye feels more comfortable again. When she looks outside the window the rainbow effect has gone. Switching on the light caused the pupil to constrict. The angle was thereby opened up again and the pressure is rapidly coming back to normal. If she had gone straight to bed the pressure would probably have reduced by morning for in sleep the pupil constricts.

The haloes seen in the above case history were an early warning of glaucoma. This housewife was lucky. No damage had been done to the optic nerve and no loss of field had taken place. Sometimes a number of sub-acute attacks of this nature occur, affecting one or both eyes. This patient was admitted to hospital and both eyes were operated on to make a small hole in the iris at the 12 o'clock position, where it is covered by the upper lid (peripheral iridectomy). This prevents the iris from bowing forward and blocking the angle. If this had not been done there would inevitably have been further sub-acute attacks which would have culminated in a full-blown attack of what is known as acute congestive glaucoma, one of the major emergencies of medicine.

Acute (congestive) glaucoma

If an attack of sub-acute glaucoma does not resolve within a few hours an attack of acute glaucoma occurs, which may well result in blindness. There are two warning symptoms: the first is pain which gradually builds up over several hours and is dull and throbbing in nature. Sometimes it is felt in the eye itself and sometimes in the brow or side of the head. It is very often associated with vomiting. The second symptom is loss of vision. This is largely due to the hazy cornea which in turn is caused by excess fluid (oedema) in the cornea. After a few hours the vision drops until the patient is barely able to count fingers held up before him. The eye is congested and angry-looking. There is no discharge from the eye, but it may water. The hazy cornea is immediately obvious if the eye with the attack is compared with the other eye. The pupil is dilated and will not constrict if a bright light is shone into it. The most important observation, however, is that of the ocular pressure. Eye surgeons are trained to estimate the level of the ocular pressure by the evidence of the finger tips, comparing the pressures of the two eyes (see Plate 3). The eye with the acute glaucoma feels as if there were a stone in the socket, whereas a gentle pressure on the normal eye will indent it.

When the pressure is measured accurately, using a tonometer, the reading will probably be around 50–60 mm Hg. There is great danger in this situation because this pressure is only a little below that in the arteries supplying blood to the interior of the eye. If the ocular pressure continues to rise it comes nearer and nearer to the point at which there is insufficient arterial pressure to keep up a flow of blood through the eye. When this happens all the tissues inside the eye are deprived of oxygen and within a few hours the sight may be permanently lost. To make matters worse the pain and anxiety of the attack often start off an acute attack in the second eye.

Acute glaucoma is a major medical emergency and urgent admission to hospital is always necessary. In order to bring down the pressure as quickly as possible two measures are adopted. The first is to constrict the pupil by means of pilocarpine drops; these are usually used in 4 per cent strength and given hourly until the pupil starts to constrict and then three-hourly until the tension has come down to within normal limits. It is worth noting here that the pilocarpine is used in this case for its effect on contracting the pupil, not to open up the pores in the trabeculum, which are of the normal size.

The other drug of great importance in the treatment of acute glaucoma is acetazolamide (Diamox). The effect of acetazolamide is to stop the formation of intra-ocular fluid. This is analogous to turning off the tap when the bath is overflowing. Diamox is usually given in tablet form, 500 mg at once and then 250 mg every six hours until the pressure is down. Diamox is also a valuable drug in the treatment of any type of secondary glaucoma. As a precautionary measure to prevent the second eye starting an acute attack it is treated with a weak solution of 1 per cent pilocarpine to ensure that the pupil is constricted.

When the immediate danger, strangulation of the blood-supply of the affected eye, has been averted, it is usual to let the eye settle for a few days before attempting surgery, as it is much easier to operate when the eye is white than when it is congested. Surgery to both eyes is always necessary after an attack of acute glaucoma, because the situation that has brought on the attack is bound to happen again.

The operation is a simple one; it is called a peripheral iridectomy. It has been described on p. 56.

8

Injuries

The eyes of reptiles and mammals are to some extent protected by the bony orbits which surround them, but they are still highly vulnerable, especially when the animal is moving among trees and undergrowth in semi-darkness. Man and monkeys have the advantage of the ability to shield their eyes with their hands; so they can move faster in conditions of low illumination, an important survival factor.

Mechanical (traumatic) are the most common injuries to the eye and will be considered first. The next most common are chemical injuries caused by corrosives (p. 65), then injuries caused by heat (p. 64), nuclear power and irradiation (p. 67), and ultraviolet light. In many of these accidents both the eyes are involved but even if only one eye is blinded the individual may have to go through life with the ever-present fear that subsequent injury or disease to the fellow eye will result in complete blindness.

Penetrating injuries

The outer tough protective coat of the eyeball formed by the cornea and sclera may be pierced or cut by a variety of sharp objects. These include missiles such as darts and arrows, cutting instruments such as scissors and knives, or high-velocity particles flying off machine tools, shattered windscreens, or from explosions.

Three hazards may accompany this type of injury. The first is damage to the delicate intra-ocular structures such as the iris, crystalline lens, and retina. The second is that micro-organisms may enter the globe and set up an intra-ocular inflammation. Finally, where missiles are involved, they may be retained inside the eye as an intra-ocular foreign body. The intra-ocular foreign body is an important type of penetrating injury; often the result of an industrial accident. It is largely preventable as most factory regulations stipulate that protective visors must be supplied and worn when workers are using lathes or other powered tools.

59

Intra-ocular foreign bodies

Another common cause of an intra-ocular foreign body is the so-called 'hammer-and-chisel' accident. The hammer is usually badly worn with a 'mushroomed' end. On striking a metal object or something less resistant such as brick or even wood, a fragment of the edge of the *hammer* flies backwards into the eye of the man using it. This means that in this type of accident the foreign body is usually steel; this is fortunate as metal shows up well on an X-ray so its exact position inside the eye can be discovered even when it is hidden by blood or buried in the tissues. Furthermore, steel particles can be removed with the aid of a magnet, making this a much easier proposition than removing a non-metallic object like stone or glass. It is always necessary to remove a steel particle from inside the eye as otherwise it slowly rusts. Iron is highly injurious to the retina and lens and eventually causes blindness months or years later (siderosis).

A corneal foreign body is a less severe injury in which the particle does not completely penetrate the globe but remains embedded on the surface of the cornea. A sub-tarsal foreign body is often blown in by the wind and lodges behind the upper lid where there is a shallow groove. Plates 4 and 5 show how corneal and sub-tarsal foreign bodies are removed: the former after instillation of one or two drops of 1 per cent amethocaine and the latter requiring no drops at all. A corneal foreign body always causes an abrasion and this is treated like any other corneal abrasion (see p. 33).

In any kind of penetrating injury the important question is: 'What injuries have been done to the structures inside the eye?' The answer will vary according to the size of the object causing the wound and the route it has taken inside the eye. No two injuries are alike, but there are some very common types of damage. A prolapsed iris often follows a corneal wound in which the anterior chamber is opened. This causes a gush of aqueous (intra-ocular fluid), and a portion of the iris is drawn up into the wound and appears on the surface as a dark knuckle of tissue between the lips of the corneal wound. The pupil is displaced by the prolapse and takes on a characteristic shape, the 'pear-shaped pupil' (Fig. 4 (a)). This requires major surgery. Sometimes the iris can be replaced but it is more usual to cut the prolapsed portion right away and although it causes a rather ugly

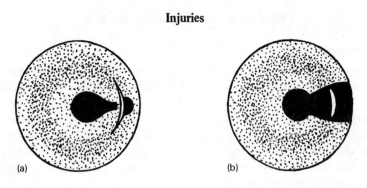

Fig. 4. Iris prolapse: (a) showing up-drawn pupil; (b) after excision of prolapse.

deformity of the pupil the sight is not seriously impaired (Fig. 4 (b)).

Injury to the crystalline lens is a very common complication of a penetrating injury. Even the smallest perforation of the lens capsule will allow the intra-ocular fluid to enter the substance of the lens and cause the lens fibres to break up and be absorbed. In the early stages this is accompanied by swelling of the lens which presses the iris against the back of the cornea so that the filtration angle is obliterated and a secondary glaucoma may result. This also happens if fragments of the softened lens obstruct the pores of the trabeculum or if adhesions form in the pupil between the lens capsule and the iris. At surgery then, it is important to remove any remains there may be of the lens, damaged iris, or vitreous which otherwise collect as a tangled mass of fibrotic material in the pupil area and which may present considerable surgical problems later on.

See also cataract (p. 40) and secondary glaucoma (p. 52).

The vitreous and retina, which are closely associated, are often involved in penetrating injuries. The pathway through the vitreous taken by the foreign body can often be tracked by the fibrotic band which subsequently forms there. This is often attached to the retina, which may be torn or even completely penetrated (through-and-through type of injury) if a projectile passes clean through the eye. A vitreous band may develop subsequently as a late complication and pull on the retina giving rise to a traction detachment (p. 21). These retino-vitreal bands can be divided surgically but traction detachments usually do badly and are often complicated by membranes of tissue forming over the macula (pre-retinal fibrosis).

Intra-ocular infections

If the eye is penetrated by a dirty implement such as a pitchfork, pus-forming micro-organisms can enter the interior of the eye and set up a severe inflammation (endophthalmitis). The eye becomes congested and angry-looking, the cornea hazy, and a yellow reflection is visible behind the pupil. Sometimes there is a greyish yellow deposit in the lower part of the anterior chamber with a horizontal fluid level (hypopyon). This is caused by pus cells settling in the lower part of the anterior chamber between the iris and the cornea.

Urgent action is needed if the eye is to be saved. The infection is combated by injection of a concentrated solution of antibiotic (such as gentamicin) under the conjunctiva, from whence it readily penetrates into the globe through the sclera. Adhesions between the cornea, iris, and damaged tissues rapidly form and give rise to raised tension and other harmful effects; these are suppressed by steroids which can also be injected under the conjunctiva. The pupil is kept dilated by atropine and similar drugs, which also help to reduce the formation of adhesions. The sub-conjunctival injections can be repeated daily for several days if necessary.

Bleeding inside the eye often complicates penetrating injuries but as it occurs more typically in non-penetrating (bruising) types of accident it will be dealt with under that heading (p. 63).

Injury to one eye may lead to the loss of sight in both. Sympathetic ophthalmia, the most dreaded complication of all, is described in the section on uveitis (p. 47).

Non-penetrating injuries

A blow from a fist or other blunt object causes the familiar black eye, a haemorrhage under the skin of the eyelid which in itself does no harm. Treatment with raw steak is outmoded: a saline pack and a fairly firm crepe bandage are more effective and very much cheaper!

All the ocular structures may suffer from a contusion injury and the easiest way to remember the various possibilities is simply to think of the eye tissues in a series of layers from the skin to the optic nerve. The bones around the eye forming the orbit are very fragile and easily broken. X-rays are often necessary to determine the extent of damage.

Injuries

A particularly troublesome type of injury is the 'blow-out' fracture in which the pressure of the blow ruptures the floor of the orbit and traps the muscles and fat under the eyeball. This prevents the eye from looking upwards. Sometimes the muscles which move the eye (extra-ocular muscles) are damaged by haemorrhage and a paretic squint (p. 73) results.

The cornea and sclera are frequently damaged. The cornea is often abraded and the eye painful (see p. 33). Occasionally the sclera ruptures and the eyeball becomes extremely soft. It is treated as for a penetrating injury.

Tears often occur at the pupil margin and injure the circular muscle surrounding the pupil with the result that it becomes permanently dilated. This is extremely inconvenient in bright light. Sometimes the iris tears at its root, causing what in effect is a second pupil, and the patient suffers from diplopia (double vision). A very important result of even a small iris tear is the formation of a *hyphaema* or collection of blood in the anterior chamber. If the eye is seen a few minutes after the injury a uniform red haze will be observed in the anterior chamber, but this soon settles by gravity and a very typical horizontal fluid level separates clear intra-ocular fluid above from red hyphaema below (Fig. 5).

A hyphaema can be seen with the naked eye and always indicates that the contusion has been severe. The patient is put to bed at home or, better, in hospital lying comfortably with the head supported until the blood absorbs. This usually takes from one to five days. Great care is taken with children as they are particularly liable to a second bleed

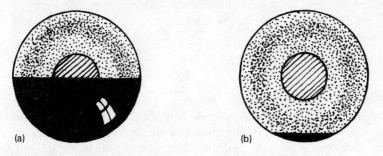

Fig. 5. Hyphaema: (a) 5 mm hyphaema; (b) one week later.

which may lead to secondary glaucoma, as the pores of the trabeculum get blocked up with red cells. Severe pain in the eye is the indication that this complication has occurred and expert help is required without delay.

The crystalline lens is sometimes jolted forcibly and its ligament torn. The eye will then be astigmatic. Secondary glaucoma and secondary cataract frequently follow. In very rare cases the lens is completely dislocated backwards into the vitreous and the eye becomes aphakic (p. 42), just as it does after a cataract operation.

The retina often tears with injury and this leads to a retinal detachment. Sometimes the tear involves a blood-vessel, and a vitreous haemorrhage results. At other times the bruising of the retina results in the accumulation of fluid (commotio-retinae) in its substance and if the macula is involved permanent damage to vision results. Less frequent are tears and haemorrhage in the choroid.

Finally, one or both optic nerves may be damaged. This is often associated with an indirect injury, for example a violent blow on the skull. In these cases the brain and optic nerves are forcibly distorted and the blood-vessels of the optic nerves, are torn. After about six weeks the optic discs become pale and atrophic and the vision is permanently impaired.

Every year hundreds of young boxers lose the sight of one or both eyes. This is not due to the 'cut eye', which is such an acute embarrassment at the time of the contest and is caused by the soft tissues of the lids being pounded against the bones surrounding the orbit. Blindness is caused by haemorrhages, secondary glaucoma, and detachment of the retina occurring up to several weeks later. These are a predictable aftermath which we consider to be justification for a ban on boxing as a sporting activity.

Burns

Burns of the eye are usually caused by 'blow-back' injuries such as petrol explosions, or gas stove explosions. The lids may suffer any degree of burn and they swell rapidly; the patient cannot open his eyes and fears he has become completely blind. Corneal abrasions are common and the pain adds to the patient's concern, moreover there are frequently multiple foreign bodies on the corneae or under the lids. These are partly due to the products of the explosion and partly to particles from the patient's charred eyelashes. The situation is often less serious than it at first seems.

The examination is made easier by instilling a pain killer, 1 per cent amethocaine, into the eyes (there is no contra-indication to this in any painful eye condition save that it is necessary to warn the patient that the pain will return in half an hour or so). Any dead skin on the lids is removed with scissors and the charred lashes clipped to the roots with scissors smeared with petroleum jelly to prevent any particles falling into the eye. The eye is irrigated with saline and any adherent foreign bodies which are left lying on the cornea or under the lids are removed (p. 60). The cornea is stained with fluorescein and the abraded areas are noted. An antibiotic ointment (chloramphenicol) is applied, and the lids are covered with tullegras and a light bandage.

Reaction to ultraviolet light also causes severe pain and mental distress. This condition is common among arc-welders working with their eyes inadequately protected by goggles, and among electricians, due to short-circuit flashes. It is the cause of 'snow-blindness' in skiers and arctic explorers and can also be caused by the mercury vapour lamps used for home sun-tanning.

Symptoms do not come on until about four hours after the exposure. There is severe pain and the lids are badly swollen. What is needed above all is reassurance, as the condition is self-limiting and passes off in a few hours. Steroid eye-drops help to reduce the reaction and so do saline compresses. There are no permanent after-effects.

Chemical injuries

Corrosive liquids, either strong alkalis such as caustic soda and ammonia, or strong acids such as nitric or hydrochloric acid (spirits of salt), are a frequent cause of industrial injury. Rather weaker concentrations of these fluids are found in household cleaning fluids. In the building trade a hazard is quicklime; in this case in the form of a powder which is mixed with sand or cement.

The chemicals can enter the eye by splashes or explosions or, in a criminal assault in which water-pistols are filled with liquid ammonia in a deliberate attempt to blind. Both eyes are frequently injured in these cases, and blindness often follows. Injuries caused by other chemically neutral fluids such as alcohol, detergents, and sprays used in agriculture are much less lethal.

Damage to the cornea is the most serious lesion caused by strong acids and alkalis. In the most severe cases the cornea becomes completely opaque and all the living cells of its substance are destroyed. In the course of a few days the cornea appears to melt away and perforates in the centre so the contents of the eyeball are infected if not expelled.

In less severe cases, although the corneal epithelium is abraded, it is at first reasonably clear. It then gradually becomes opaque and is invaded by new-formed vessels from the sclera. A uveitis is set up and this causes severe pain and congestion which often lasts for months. The eye may also become glaucomatous and develop a secondary cataract. When, and only when, these secondary effects of corrosive burns have been controlled and the eye is quiet again, the opaque cornea may be grafted; however, the graft is frequently rejected by damaged tissues.

Besides the damage to the cornea the conjunctiva, especially the lower fornix, which is the narrow crevice formed by the back of the lower lid and the eyeball, is often affected. The corrosive runs down into the fornix and denudes both sides of the crevice so that the eyeball and lower lid stick together in a firm scar which prevents the free movements of the globe. This can be dealt with surgically. A more serious result of a chemical burn, however, is that small glands which lie within the membrane of the conjunctiva are destroyed. These secrete tears and mucous and they are essential to the health of the conjunctiva and cornea. The resulting drying of the eye leads to xerosis (p. 85) and the condition is extremely difficult to alleviate.

Emergency treatment is essential in these injuries. Seconds count! The all important thing is to dilute the corrosive by *any* means to hand. Put the victim's head under a tap, plunge it into a bucket of water, or douse the eye with coca-cola or any watery fluid available. There are theoretical antidotes such as sodium bicarbonate for acids and boric acid for alkalis, but prolonged irrigation of the eye with normal saline is as good as anything. If the corrosive has not been diluted it will have already done irreparable harm by the time the victim reaches the hospital or clinic. Most chemical burns of the eye need hospitalization, which may be prolonged.

Lime burns of the eye differ from those due to other corrosives in that the powdered lime cakes into firm plaques which adhere to the conjunctiva, especially under the upper lid. These are removed by anaesthetizing the conjunctiva with 1 per cent amethocaine drops and picking off the plaques with fine forceps. The eye is then irrigated copiously with 0.4 per cent sodium edathamil (EDTA). A very effective emergency treatment in the old days, when lime-burns were much more common, was for a workmate to pass his tongue over the eyeball and under the lids. Not for the squeamish, but many an eye was saved thereby.

Radiation injuries

The eye can be damaged by any form of radiant energy. When the eye itself is being irradiated to treat retinoblastoma or malignant melanoma the radiation injuries are the lesser of the two evils and therefore acceptable. The eye may also be damaged during the irradiation of malignant tumours of the skin and nasal sinuses lying close to it. Occasionally radiologists and radiographers become the accidental victims of imperfectly shielded X-ray apparatus. There were hundreds of eye radiation injuries following the atom bomb explosions in Japan.

The tissue of the eye most likely to be affected is the crystalline lens, but the cornea also may be damaged. The lens, as might be expected, forms a cataract; but this does not happen immediately. For months there is no apparent damage but then fine opacities develop in the cortex and then a more defined, denser, cataract forms in the centre of the back layers of the lens (posterior sub-capsular cataract) where it does most damage to sight. The cataract may take years to mature and it often 'stops in its tracks'; this is especially true of the atom bomb cataracts. These cataracts are treatable by surgery on the same general lines as has been described elsewhere (p. 42).

The cornea is usually damaged only when it has been exposed to a high dose of irradiation, for example when it has been in the direct pathway of an X-ray beam. The main lesions are a series of minute erosions of the corneal epithelium. These are very painful and may take many months to clear.

Blindness and visual handicap: the facts

High-voltage electric shocks sometimes result in cataracts very similar to those caused by radiant energy. They take months to become apparent and are usually incomplete.

9

Refractive error and squint

Refractive errors

Man's eyes are designed for seeing things at a distance: things which may mean the difference between life and death such as a herd of mammoth miles away or a landfall from a tiny coracle drifting in the ocean. A man gifted with perfect eyes focuses a distant object exactly on the retina. Rays of light from a distant object are parallel until they meet the cornea, when they are sharply bent by its curved surface. They are bent again by the crystalline lens and thus brought to a focus exactly on the retina in much the same way that the rays of the sun can be focused to a spot of intense light by a burning glass. This ideal condition of exact focus of distant objects is called emmetropia.

If the length of an eye is shorter than the normal one inch (25 mm) the bending of the rays of light will not be fully effective so the image formed on the retina will be blurred. This condition is long sight or hypermetropia. It does not mean that the eye sees further than a normal eye; it just sees relatively better for distant objects than for near. Conversely if an eye is longer than the normal, as in short sight, or myopia, the image of a distant object is formed in front of the retina and again the image is blurred.

A third way in which a distant object cannot be brought to a focus on the retina is when the eye suffers from astigmatism. This is caused by the fact that the curve of the cornea is not uniform like the surface of a sphere, but more curved in one direction than another like the surface of the back of a spoon. This distorts the image. These three conditions, hypermetropia, myopia, and astigmatism, are called refractive errors and they can be corrected by suitable lenses.

In order to focus on near objects in emmetropia and hypermetropia the rays of light must be bent even more sharply to obtain the image on the retina: this mechanism is called focusing or accommodation. It is performed without conscious effort on our behalf by a ring of muscles inside the eye which relax the suspensory ligament of the lens and make it more convex. In consequence the bending of the rays of light is more marked.

In myopia simply by getting nearer to the object, or bringing the object nearer to the eye, brings its image exactly on to the retina.

When a person is aged between 40 and 45 another condition develops: presbyopia or the sight of aging. It occurs because the crystalline lens becomes stiffer with age and the muscles cannot alter its curvature as readily as in youth. It is for this reason that some time after the age of 40 people have to have a stronger pair of glasses for reading. This addition for reading has gradually to be increased until the age of 60. Some short-sighted people have the advantage here for they can often read simply by taking off their distance glasses. There are radical differences in the degree of presbyopia present at any given age. People from the Indian sub-continent usually require a higher presbyopic correction at any given age than those of the same age in north-west Europe.

Refractive errors can be corrected by placing a spectacle lens of the right strength in front of the eye. A lens may be convex (+), in which case parallel rays of light will be brought to a focus on the retina in a hypermetropic eye. In a myopic eye in which parallel rays come to a focus in front of the retina a concave (−) spectacle lens will cause the light rays to diverge before entering the eye and thus bring them to a focus exactly on the retina.

The strength or bending power of a spectacle lens is measured by a unit called a dioptre. The higher the dioptre number the stronger the lens. A man who is myopic and can just see the top letter of the test types will require a concave lens of −3.0 dioptres to correct his vision to 6/6, so that he can read the bottom line of the chart. We say that the eye has −3.0 dioptres of myopia. Again, after the age of 60 a presbyopic person will need an additional strength of (convex) lens of between +2.50 and 3.0 dioptres for reading. This is called his presbyopic correction. In astigmatism, if the horizontal lines of an object are in focus the vertical ones are not, and vice versa. This error can be corrected by a special cylindrical lens, which is like a round glass rod cut lengthways. These cylindrical lenses can be added to those needed to correct other refractive errors.

Refractive error and squint

Myopia

Hypermetropia, astigmatism, and presbyopia do not in themselves cause any ocular diseases but the same is not true of myopia. In the higher degrees of this conditon there may be ocular complications which result in impaired vision or even blindness. There are two forms of myopia, a benign condition called simple myopia and a less common but more severe form called high or malignant myopia. In both forms of myopia the eyeball is lengthened, and the condition is present in both eyes. The condition often runs in families and the Japanese and Jewish people are particularly prone to the condition. The optics and the use of minus lenses to focus the light on the retina instead of in front of it have already been described. Myopia is measured by the strength of the minus lens required to do this. In simple myopia the strength of the minus lens required is less than —6.0 dioptres. In high myopia, however, the strength of the lens needed is over —6.0 dioptres and may be up to a —20-dioptre lens or even —30; this means that the globe has elongated 7–10 mm and the patient will have noticeably protruding eyes.

Simple myopia usually starts between the ages of 10 and 18 and the power of the correcting lenses has to be gradually increased until the age of 22 or so. Apart from the difficulty in seeing distant objects there is little real disability and complications are rare.

In high myopia the condition starts younger and the minus correction has to be gradually increased into middle life. Several complications are found in this condition, probably due to the mechanical stretching of the sclera of the back half of the globe. It may be that the sclera is weaker than normal and unable to resist the intra-ocular pressure, which gives perfectly normal readings. Although the sclera, which is made of tough tendon-like tissue, can stretch, the retina, which is made of nervous tissue, and the choroid, which is composed almost entirely of blood-vessels cannot, and both these structures may suffer.

As we have already seen (p. 22) a high myope is liable to retinal detachment. The reason for this is not known for certain but not infrequently one finds areas of retinal degeneration near the periphery of myopic fundi, and these are often the sites where retinal holes form. These myopic detachments are treated in the same way as other types of retinal detachments. As there is an inbuilt weakness in myopic retinae a high myope should never engage in boxing, wrestling, weight-lifting, or field games in which hard falls are to be expected.

In high myopia it is quite common for the stretched choroid to atrophy. When this occurs the choroidal vessels slowly disappear and the ophthalmoscope shows patches of white sclera where the choroid is missing. These atrophic patches are blind areas as the rods and cones of the retina have lost their blood-supply. As time goes on the patches enlarge and coalesce and if the central area is involved macular vision is lost. This is sometimes associated with small retinal haemorrhages called Fuch's spots.

The vitreous gel is also affected in high myopia. Instead of filling the interior of the globe it retracts away from the retina (vitreous retraction) and the space between them is filled with intra-ocular fluid. Sometimes the jelly disrupts and denser parts float about in the more fluid parts like water-weeds, causing the effect of floating shadows or simply 'floaters'. These are not in themselves of any very serious import but they are annoying to the patient (see also vitreous floaters, p. 37).

A final complication of high myopia is that there is an increased tendency to cataract in this condition.

Squint

Many people who have only one eye manage perfectly well in life even though they often want to do things that most others have difficulty in doing with two. Wiley Post, the pioneer American airman, for example, flew round the world solo with his single eye.

What then is the advantage of having two eyes? First and foremost it is a considerable help in the assessment of the distance of objects and their exact position in relation to us. You will find that you can touch the right-hand upper corner of this page more easily and accurately with both eyes open than with either closed. This ability to use both eyes together is called binocular or stereoscopic vision. The stereoscopic world is a three-dimensional world obtained by a simple optical trick. It depends on the fact that as the eyes are about three inches apart the image of the world that we obtain from each eye is slightly different and these two images are 'built-up' by the brain to form a solid single picture.

Linked closely with stereopsis are the movements of the eyes. Both must be lined up on the same object otherwise it appears double. The ideal state is when the eyes are aligned on a distant object, when each one is looking perfectly straight ahead. When his gaze is directed to an object nearer to him the observer has to converge his eyes so that the images still fall on the foveae. If the object is brought nearer and nearer to the eyes they converge even more strongly until finally, the strain of keeping up binocular vision is too great and it 'breaks-down'. When this happens one or other eye does the seeing and the other drifts outwards.

An eye which deviates either inwards or outwards from the position it should hold when viewing an object at any distance is said to have a squint or heterotropia. This can occur for one of three reasons. First the eye may be diseased so that the retinal image is defective or indeed, absent. This is called a *sensory* squint. The poor retinal image may result from a number of causes from a deformity present at birth to a retinal degeneration appearing in old age. Binocular vision requires two good images and if one is imperfect there is no mental stimulus to 'fuse' the two images and the eye with the poorer vision simply wanders off. In children the bad eye usually turns inwards (convergent squint), and in adults outwards (divergent squint).

The second reason for a squint is a paralysis of one or more of the ocular muscles. Six muscles enable each eye to move in any direction, and they are 'yoked' by a complicated nervous mechanism so that both eyes move together in the same direction. This arrangement is easily disturbed by injury, swellings in the vicinity, or by diseases of the nervous system such as meningitis and multiple sclerosis. These are called *paretic* squints and they have a very important symptom, diplopia or double vision, which is more marked when the patient is looking in the direction in which the paralysed muscle would normally exert its strongest pull.

The third reason for a squint is the absence of the smooth co-ordination between accommodation (focusing) and convergence. This is the most common type of squint, especially in children and called *accommodative* squint. It is also called concomitant squint as it is present to the same degree all the time and does not alter with the direction of gaze as does a paretic squint.

Children are usually long-sighted (hypermetrophic) at birth so in order to look at things close to they have to over-accommodate. This over-accommodation can cause over-convergence and hence a convergent squint. The opposite is the case in myopes. Here there is less stimulus to accommodate as the eye is already in focus for near objects. Under-accommodation then leads to a lessened stimulus to converge and the eye tends to take up a divergent position.

Suppression and amblyopia

If the eyes squint there is a double image of everything. A child very soon learns how to overcome this difficulty. It uses one eye only, usually the one with the smaller refractive error as this has the clearest image. The image obtained by the other (squinting) eye is ignored. This is known as suppression and is quite easy. Riflemen, for example, usually keep both eyes open when shooting but concentrate on the target with one eye only and take no notice of (or suppress) the other.

Suppression in squint, although a solution to the immediate problem of diplopia, is harmful as the brain eventually refuses to accept the image from the squinting eye which becomes amblyopic or lazy and suffers a marked loss of vision. The eye itself, it must be stressed, is perfectly normal in every respect. Suppression can lead to blindness in the squinting eye. But an amblyopic eye is very easy to treat. The good eye is covered with plaster in the very young or by an opaque occluder in older children, making them look only through the squinting eye. In a short time, and the younger the child the quicker the result, the vision will return to the squinting eye. But the child must not even have a peep with the good eye in the meantime!

Treatment

The rationale of the treatment of squint is as follows:
1. A careful examination of the eyes is made to ensure that there is no disease present.
2. The refraction must be worked out and any necessary glasses ordered.
3. The 'good' eye is occluded (the patient is now under supervision by the orthoptist).
4. When the vision in the squinting eye has been restored and the child can fix with either eye it is possible, using an instrument known as a synoptophore, to train him to use both eyes together, even though a squint may still be present.

5. When binocular vision has been established surgery is usually necessary to put the eyes into alignment.
6. Further orthoptic treatment is given to make the desire for binocular vision even stronger.

An old wives' tale which dies hard and leads to much loss of vision is that the child's eye will get straight in time without any treatment. This is sometimes true but the sad fact is that it will probably be a worthless amblyopic one. Squints must be treated just as soon as they are apparent.

10

Visual pathways

Images of the world around us are formed on our retinae, and the interpretation of what we are seeing is done by a specialized part of the brain called the occipital (visual) cortex. This is situated under the most prominent part of the back of the skull or occiput. A long, cable-like nervous pathway connects the eyes to the occipital cortex. It is called the visual pathway. It has a long distance to travel in the centre of the brain and there are many places and many ways in which the nerve fibres of which it is composed can be damaged.

Anatomy

The visual pathway on each side consists of the optic nerve, the chiasma (crossing), the optic tract, the optic radiation, and the occipital (visual) cortex (Fig. 6). The optic nerve runs from the optic disc backwards to the chiasma and carries all the fibres of the retina from that eye. The chiasma is a band-shaped structure lying between the brain above and the pituitary gland below. It is here that the optic nerves meet and the nasal fibres from each retina cross to the other side.

The optic tract and optic radiations fan out backwards in the brain substance to the occipital cortex and consist of the temporal retinal fibres of the same side and the nasal fibres of the opposite side. The occipital cortex of each side lies close to its fellow. There is a fissure in the brain tissue called the calcarine sulcus and it is around this that the visual sensations are received.

Field loss in visual pathway defects

The relationship of the field of vision to any part of the visual pathways is easy to understand if one knows some simple facts.
1. Each retina divides vertically into two halves, an inner (nasal) and an outer (temporal) half (Fig. 6).

Visual pathways

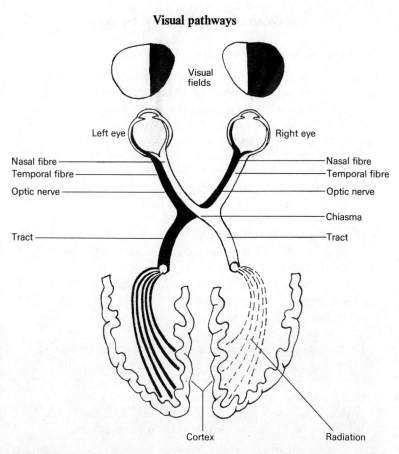

Fig. 6. The optic pathways.

2. Because the retinal images are reversed we see the temporal (outer) half of each visual field with the inner (nasal) half of each retina and vice versa.
3. The fibres of the *temporal* halves of the retinae go to the cortex of the *same* side whereas the fibres of the *nasal* halves cross in the chiasma and go to the cortex of the *opposite* side.
4. Therefore the right cortex receives both the left halves of the fields of vision (i.e. one from each eye) and the left cortex the images from the two right halves of the fields of vision.

Blindness and visual handicap: the facts

Conditions affecting the optic nerve

The optic nerve is about two inches long and runs from the back of the globe (where it can be seen with the ophthalmoscope as the optic disc) to the optic chiasma, which lies in the cranial cavity just below the brain. Many conditions can affect the nerve in this course. The fibres may be compressed by tumours or localized expansions of the blood-vessels (aneurysms), injured in blows to the skull (pp. 64, 96), or patches of inflammation or degeneration may develop along its course, as in multiple sclerosis. All these conditions will give a visual field defect on the same side of the compression, injury, or inflammation. There will also probably be an impairment of the normal reflex constriction of the pupil when a light is shone into the affected eye. This is because the nerve fibres which serve this pupil reaction travel to the brain alongside the visual fibres in the optic nerve.

When the nerve fibres are damaged they atrophy, or die, for nerve tissue, unlike many other tissue, cannot regenerate. This death is apparent on examining the optic disc, which loses its normal pink colour and becomes white (optic atrophy).

Cerebral tumours sometimes cause the intracranial pressure to rise, and this may cause swelling and congestion of the disc called papill-oedema. This does not in itself cause loss of vision unless it has been present for several months. The disc may also show swelling if a patch of inflammation lies near it (optic neuritis) and this is always associated with a central field defect and loss of vision (central scotoma).

Chiasma to cortex

The chiasma lies above the pituitary gland in the base of the skull. The pituitary is a common site of tumour formation. As the tumour enlarges it presses up to the central part of the chiasma where the nasal fibres cross. These nasal fibres carry visual impulses from the temporal visual fields so the effect on vision is like a horse wearing blinkers – side vision is reduced or absent. I can recall a patient in whom this condition was diagnosed as he was the middle man of a trio of cyclists and he kept banging into his two fellow riders!

The optic tracts which carry the visual fibres to the mid-brain may also be involved by tumours and by occlusions of the blood-vessels. Each tract carries the temporal fibres from the same side and the nasal fibres from the other so either the right or left halves of the fields of vision are defective. This is called a homonymous hemianopia of the right or left side. The visual fibres finally pass in the optic radiations to the visual cortex in the occipital part of the brain. Damage to the fibres in these regions is usually caused by occlusions of the cerebral arteries, by aneurysms, or by tumours. All these result in hemianopic fields similar to those which have been described above in damage to tracts.

11

Disorders of the conjunctiva, eyelids, and tear-producing apparatus

Three structures are concerned with protecting the globe and keeping the front parts of the eye moist: the conjunctiva, the lids, and the lacrymal apparatus which is concerned with tear production. The three are closely linked and are often called the ocular adnexae.

Structure and function of the conjunctiva

The conjunctiva is a thin, transparent membrane which covers the back surfaces of the lids and the front part of the sclera (the white of the eye). It has its own system of blood-vessels which can be seen with the naked eye, and numerous microscopic glands which secrete mucus and some of the tears. It also covers the front of the cornea, but here its structure is entirely different. It consists of a very frail layer of transparent tissue called the corneal epithelium. This has been described with the cornea (p. 31), of which it forms an integral part.

The main function of the conjunctiva is to lubricate the front of the eyeball so it can move smoothly behind the lids. If the conjunctiva becomes dry because of lack of tears, protrusion of the globe (proptosis), or paralysis of the lid muscles the cornea and conjunctiva rapidly become lustreless and opaque (see xerosis, p. 66, 105).

Conjunctivitis

Conjunctivitis is an inflammation of the conjunctiva. There are three types: the first is *bacterial* conjunctivitis, and this is the most common type. It can be due to a number of different kinds of organisms which may cause disease in other parts of the body. Examples of these are staphylococci which cause boils and styes; streptococci which sometimes cause septicaemia; pneumococci, which cause pneumonia, and many others. Of special importance in ophthalmology are gonococci which cause gonorrhoea in the adult and which may cause blindness

80

in babies (ophthalmia neonatorum), and pseudomonas infection which is deadly to the eye once it gains entry.

The second type is *allergic* conjunctivitis. Many people are born with various allergies and some suddenly develop a sensitivity to something that they may have been in contact with for years such as hair sprays, primulas, or certain foods. The conjunctiva can be affected by the reaction.

Lastly, conjunctivitis may be due to a *viral* infection and, worldwide, the most common of these is trachoma, a chronic blinding disease (p. 100) with an estimated 500 million sufferers. A similar but less virulent virus is the TRIC virus which causes a disease with a much shorter and more benign course.

Symptoms and treatment

Bacterial conjunctivitis is not painful but sometimes causes a gritty feeling. The sight is not affected. The hall-mark is a discharge which is very variable in degree. There is a velvety redness of the conjunctiva which is seen to best advantage when the lower lid is pulled down to expose the lower fornix. The patient is warned that he may transfer the infection to others by unclean hands, or by towels, and facecloths. The discharge is cultured in the laboratory and the type of organism is identified. The pathologist is also able to recommend the most effective antibiotic for any particular case. Sometimes this is not necessary and treatment by a 'broad-spectrum' antibiotic (which means one effective against a wide range of bacteria) is used. Examples of these are chloramphenicol or gentamicin used as drops every two hours and the dosage gradually reduced over 6–10 days. If the treatment is stopped too soon the condition is liable to relapse. The eye is never padded but the patient is usually more comfortable wearing dark glasses. Ophthalmia neonatorum is treated by intensive antibiotic therapy: one drop a minute for 30 minutes and every 5 minutes for the next hour: and hourly for the rest of the first day. Sulphonamides are given by mouth.

In allergic conjunctivitis the eyes itch and the lids are swollen. Discharge is scanty. A search is made for the sensitizing agent, often with a negative result. Antihistamines are usually the most effective treatment and short-term local steroid treatment can be given only under specialist supervision.

81

Viral conjunctivitis is usually self-limiting and local sulphonamide treatment may be effective. For the treatment of trachoma see p. 101.

Pterygium

A pterygium is a fleshy, tongue-shaped pad involving both the cornea and conjunctiva and starting from where the two meet (the limbus) at the inner side of the 'whites' of one or both eyes. It grows very slowly across the cornea as a well-defined area looking rather like the wing of an insect; a number of blood-vessels run in it. It takes years before sight is threatened, when the central part of the cornea is invaded. The condition is mostly found in dusty cloudless areas of the world and apart from the obvious element of chronic irritation the cause is unknown. Most cases slowly (over years) advance up to 3 or 4 mm across the cornea and then gradually regress with the accompanying vessels becoming smaller. If the pterygium nears the pupil and threatens vision it can be removed surgically. Very occasionally pterygium forms on the outer side of the limbus.

Structure and function of the eyelids

The upper and lower lids form the first line of defence of the eye. They consist of a rigid plate of cartilage, the tarsal plate, which has in front of it the skin and a muscle called the orbicularis which enables us to screw up our eyes. Behind the tarsal plate is the conjunctiva of the lid.

The normal blinking, which takes place every few seconds, keeps the cornea lubricated and moist. In addition there is the sudden involuntary (reflex) blinking which occurs as a response to danger and saves our eyes from countless injuries.

Disorders of the eyelids

Styes are boils forming in the lash follicles. They are caused by staphylococci which multiply in the depths of the follicle and form pus. This eventually discharges on the lid margin at or near the opening of the offending follicle. Styes rarely need incision but they do require liberal

82

applications of antibiotic ointments to prevent similar infections of neighbouring follicles.

Miebomian cysts (chalazia) are swellings of the lids caused by the distention of glands which lie in the cartilage of the tarsal plates. These glands secrete an oily material which waterproofs the margin of the lids and prevents the tears running over the cheeks. The glands, of which there are some twenty or so in each lid open by a series of minute holes just behind the lashes. If one of these gets blocked by the hardening of its own secretion, a small swelling about the size of a pea forms in the lid. It frequently becomes infected and is then easily mistaken for a stye. However, a stye will resolve in a few days but a cyst nearly always requires to be opened surgically before it clears up. This is done under local anaesthesia and when the cyst has been incised the contents are removed by a curette, a small sharp-edged spoon. This operation must have been common in Roman times for there are many examples of their curettes in the museums.

Blepharitis is an inflammation of the lid margin. The most usual form is squamous blepharitis in which small white scales of dried skin lie between the lashes. It is usually associated with dandruff of the scalp and the treatment is directed towards this. A more severe form is ulcerative blepharitis in which crusts of dried pus form along the lid margins. It is often found in debilitated communities and requires prolonged treatment by antibiotics.

Trichiasis is a condition which may follow ulcerative blepharitis and is common in the later stages of trachoma (p. 101). The inflammations distort the lash follicles so that instead of sweeping forward in graceful curves they grow in an irregular manner like a row of pea sticks. Some grow inward and rub against the epithelium of the cornea with the result that it becomes ulcerated and scarred. Trichiasis can be corrected quite easily by simple plastic operations.

Herpes ophthalmicus

Herpes zoster, or shingles, is due to a virus which invades the nuclei of sensory nerves in the central nervous system. The virus is the same as that which causes chicken-pox and the patient (who is usually past middle life) has frequently been in recent contact with a case. In fact it is a 'second infection' from the virus; instead of getting chicken-pox again the patient, whose tissues are 'hypersensitive' has a skin reaction. This is often on the trunk but sometimes on the face. The areas of skin involved correspond to the sensory nerve distribution and the skin itself forms a series of small blisters which resemble the more widespread pustules of ordinary chicken-pox.

The sensory nerve which supplies the eye, the lids, and the scalp up to the top of the head is the ophthalmic nerve, one of the three branches of the trigeminal nerve which is the sensory nerve of the rest of the face. When this nerve becomes involved in a zoster inflammation the first sign is a tenderness over the skin of the forehead and it is not for two or three days that there is any evidence of a rash. When this arrives the diagnosis is no longer in doubt. At this stage it is important to be able to tell if the eye is going to be involved. If it is there will be a few little vesicles on the side of the nose on the affected side.

The most common eye lesions in herpes ophthalmicus are keratitis and uveitis. It is often several days before there are positive signs of either and a close watch is kept. Treatment of either keratitis (which may be in the form of superficial or deep keratitis) or uveitis has already been described (pp. 33 and 47); both are potentially serious conditions which may result in loss of sight in the affected eye.

The skin rash is very variable in its severity but the vesicles always become infected and form crusted plaques over the lids, forehead, and scalp, often taking weeks to clear and leaving pitted scars when they do so. They are best treated by liberal applications of antibiotic ointment.

A further complication which may last for months or even years is a particularly intractable pain (post-herpetic neuralgia).

Structure and function of the lacrymal apparatus

The tears are vitally important to the health of the eyes. They are mainly formed in a gland, the lacrymal gland, situated in the upper and outer part of the orbit. The tears pass by a series of little ducts to the upper fornix of the conjunctiva and from there they flow over the cornea and front surface of the globe. In addition to the main tear flow there are minute glands in the conjunctiva which produce both mucus and tears.

Disorders of the conjunctiva, eyelids, and tear-producing apparatus

Tears flow from the eye to the back of the nose (the reason we sniff when we cry) through narrow tubes called the lacrymal passages. These passages start at the puncta. These are two small holes at the inner ends of both the upper and lower lid margins and are visible to the naked eye. The tears flow into the puncta by syphoning and are carried by two narrow tubes, the canaliculi, into a pocket-like recess whch lies behind the place where the inner ends of the lids meet. This recess is called the lacrymal sac and from here they are carried by another narrow tube, the lacrymal duct, which finally delivers the tears to the back of the nose.

Wet and dry eyes

If there is an obstruction to the flow of tears in any part of the lacrymal passages a watering eye (epiphora) will result. This may happen in young babies if there is a delay in the formation of a hollow canaliculus; it usually opens eventually but if there is a delay of over nine months it may be necessary to open it surgically by passing a fine probe.

Obstructions in the lacrymal sac, duct, or nose may cause epiphora and these can often be relieved by syringing the passages or probing. Sometimes the puncta are too small, or sagging lids may pull them from the eye, in which case the normal syphoning of the conjunctival sac cannot take place. These conditions can be rectified by enlarging the puncta surgically if they are too small or moving them into the right position by means of a small plastic operation. If the obstruction is in the lacrymal duct it can be by-passed by a plastic operation in which the lacrymal sac can be sutured to the lining membrane of the nose (dacryocystorhinostomy, or DCR for short).

Dry eyes may be much more serious than wet ones and a dryness of the conjunctiva occurs in many conditions. Sometimes a normal quantity of tears is produced but they evaporate too easily, as happens when the eyeball is exposed when the globe is pushed forward (proptosis as in thyroid disease) or when there is a paralysis of the lids (lagophthalmos). Again, following inflammations such as trachoma the conjunctival glands may be destroyed, and there is a lack of mucus. Vitamin A deficiency, causing xerosis, is another example (see p. 104) and so is Sjögren's disease in which there is dryness of the eyes, joints, mouth, and larynx. To some extent these conditions can be alleviated by 'artificial tears' a solution which is like real tears in composition and applied by dropper every few hours. It is sometimes necessary to protect the cornea from exposure by suturing the lids together and thus partially or fully to close the eye (tarsorrhaphy) for a period of several months.

12

Blindness in children

Some 200 children under the age of 15 are registered blind every year in England and Wales and four times that number in the United States. Half of them are blind at birth.

The most common cause of blindness in the young is a fault in the development of the whole eye or in certain parts of it. The cells of the embryo reproduce themselves in a regular pre-determined manner as though a 'blue-print' were being followed and in most cases this is adhered to very strictly. However, certain chromosomes of the dividing cells may become damaged in fetal life by virus infections or other harmful agents or, less frequently, the 'blue-print' itself may develop a fault and in this case the defect is passed on from generation to generation (a genetic defect).

Most of these developmental errors are present at birth, but sometimes the defect does not show itself until well into adult life. An extreme example of this is senile macular degeneration (p. 17) which is often familial and does not appear until the sixth or seventh decade.

The development of the eye

The eye starts to form very early in the life of the embryo, about the fourth week after conception. At that stage two hollow tubes grow outwards from the brain towards the side of the head. These tubes are called the optic vesicles and are destined to form the retinae. As the tubes get near the surface the ends expand and become cup-shaped. Each cup encloses a piece of skin which detaches itself from the surface; this is the early crystalline lens.

The cells of the outer layer of the cup eventually form the pigment cell layer, and the cells of the inner layer multiply to form all the other cells and nerve fibres of the retina. The nerve fibres must eventually run to the brain, and they are enfolded by the optic nerve (which is the stalk of the cup) by a process in which the cup invaginates (turns itself inside out). This causes a notch in both the cup and the nerve and is known as the fetal fissure. These three structures, the cup, the lens, and the fissure are all well formed by the end of the second month of intra-uterine life and are the most important lines of the 'blue-print'.

In the third and fourth months the crystalline lens changes from a hollow sphere to a solid one (the nucleus-to-be) and then increases in size: laminated lens fibres grow in front of and behind it to form the lens cortex. As we have seen before (p. 39) the oldest parts of the lens are those right in the middle. At the same time the optic cup becomes surrounded by blood-vessels which are destined to form the choroid, ciliary body, and iris of the uveal tract. Later again the primitive eye acquires its firm protective coat; the cornea and sclera. Last to form are the vitreous gel, the suspensory ligament of the lens, and the anterior chamber. All these structures are developed by the sixth month of fetal life.

At each and every stage normal development may be altered or arrested. As these developmental errors are the major cause of blindness in children they will be dealt with first.

Developmental defects

If the optic vesicle fails to develop normally in one or both eyes the whole eye may be absent or represented by a small cyst in the socket (anophthalmos). In these cases the lids are usually present but are very small. A more common defect is that the eyeball is smaller than normal (micophthalmos). Sometimes these eyes see normally in childhood but as the patient gets older and the lens becomes larger there is insufficient room inside the eye and the iris is pushed towards the cornea, causing a secondary glaucoma. Again, these microphthalmic eyes often have other defects like cataract and the chances of saving the sight by any form of surgery are slender.

If the development is arrested at the time that the fetal fissure is forming, a notch, which represents it, is found in the tissues which surround the cup. The most common defect is a coloboma (notch) of the iris. This appears as a pear-shaped pupil with the notch facing downward. It often causes little interference of vision. Sometimes the notch involves the choroid, which may be missing over a large area of the fundus in the sector which represents the defect; again, the optic disc may be involved. In these cases the vision is usually poor.

The iris may be missing entirely or be represented by a small frill of tissue, a condition called aniridia. It is nearly always present in both eyes and has a strong tendency to run in families. It gives the appearance of a very large pupil with complete absence of iris colour. As there is no pupil to control the amount of light entering the eye there are difficulties in bright light. Because of the malformation in the region of the filtration angle glaucoma is liable to develop and this is sometimes delayed until middle life; periodic monitoring of the intra-ocular pressure is required.

Glaucoma

Glaucoma takes a different form in children from that in adults. It is usually found in both eyes and is present at birth. Milder cases sometimes do not become evident until a year or so, and in these cases the effects tend to be more marked on one side than the other.

The cornea and sclera in babies are very elastic and the effect of raised pressure is to cause the eyeball to enlarge. This appearance is called buphthalmos or 'ox eye'. It is usually caused by a faulty development of the filtration angle. Normally the cornea and iris are loosely united by cellular tissue until about the fifth month of fetal life. Then a cleft appears forming the anterior chamber and at the same time separating iris and cornea. It is when this intervening tissue lying in the filtration angle fails to be absorbed that the entrance to the pores in the trabeculum is blocked and the pressure rises.

In severe cases the infant has a marked cloudiness of the corneae. The expansion of the eyeball as a whole also causes the cornea to increase in size so instead of being some 10 mm or so in diameter as it normally is at birth it measures 12 mm or more. Cupping and atrophy of the optic disc are later signs. The baby is distressed, cannot bear the light (photophobia), and is constantly rubbing its watering eyes. Sometimes when he is deeply asleep, particularly after a feed, it is possible to make quite a detailed examination including a fundus exploration without any sedation at all. However a general anaesthetic will be required if tonometry is to be carried out.

The treatment is surgical. Its object is to promote the flow of intra-ocular fluid from the anterior chamber to Schlemm's canal. This can be done under direct vision through the cornea by removing the tissue blocking the trabeculum. An instrument called an operating gonioscope (angle viewer) is used and the tissue removed by cutting it away with a sharp knife. More recently another method has been evolved whereby Schlemm's canal is opened from the outside of the globe and an instrument slid along its course, breaking its wall into the anterior chamber and thereby gaining direct drainage into the canal (trabeculotomy). Unfortunately the success rate of these operations in children is very much lower than in adult glaucoma.

Cataract

Mention has already been made of developmental cataracts, or congenital cataracts as they are sometimes loosely termed (p. 40); several types which occur in early post-natal life also deserve mention. The first of these is lamellar cataract. In this condition a layer of opaque lens fibres lying between a clear nucleus is formed during fetal life, and another clear zone of variable width is laid down subsequently. The opacity is in some cases related to defective calcium metabolism; the child may suffer convulsions and defective enamel in the permanent teeth. In most cases there is no clue as to the cause.

Galactocaemic cataract is extremely rare but worthy of note because galactocaemia is treatable by medical means, and the eye signs may be of considerable help in making a diagnosis. Without treatment galacto-caemia is fatal.

The cataracts form in the first few weeks of life and have a very characteristic appearance, rather like a drop of oil suspended in the crystalline lens. The baby is obviously ill and failing to thrive. It will not take its feeds properly and the liver becomes enlarged. Mental retardation follows later.

The condition is due to the child having an inability to convert a sugar called galactose, which is formed by the digestion of milk, into glucose, which is the form in which it is used for energy in the body.

The galactose, instead of being utilized by the body, accumulates in the tissues. Once the diagnosis is made the treatment is simple: the baby must have no more milk, human or otherwise, and be reared on synthetic foods.

Cataracts are found in children suffering from thyroid deficiency (cretinism) and also in mongols (Down's disease). These cataracts are composed of numerous opaque dots scattered in the cortex of the lens and this is a sure sign that they have occurred in the postnatal years. No treatment for the eye condition is necessary as the sight is rarely affected to any degree. Diabetic cataract does rarely occur in children but it is important as sometimes the cataract matures very rapidly in a matter of weeks. With surgery the outlook is good.

Retinal blindness

Retinal aplasia (Leber's congenital retinal aplasia) is a familial condition in which the infant is apparently blind at birth. If the fundus is examined in the first few months of life it may appear quite normal and it is often thought that the baby's blindness has been caused by birth injury. However, if electrodiagnostic tests are done, even at an early age, they will reveal an abnormal response to light stimulus. Apart from the blindness the child is quite normal and if the fundus is examined after another two or three years the appearance shows a marked change, with scattered deposits of pigment and narrowing of the retinal vessels. Optic nerve atrophy comes later; the diagnosis is then obvious. There is no treatment.

Retinal aplasia is akin to retinitis pigmentosa (p. 19), in that it is an abiotrophy. In these conditions the tissues appear to have formed normally but sooner or later they fail to function properly as though they do not have the vitality of the normal tissues and suffer an early death. There are a number of conditions which are variations on the same theme. Retinitis pigmentosa is the most common but is not often diagnosed before the age of five.

A tragic but fortunately rare condition which causes blindness in babies is Tay-Sachs disease. The condition is most common in Jewish families. The child develops normally until about seven months and then it fails to thrive. It is listless, takes no interest in its surroundings, and fails to recognize familiar faces. Fits are frequent and there are long periods of coma. The baby is usually blind by its first birthday and for the next year it ekes out a pitiable existence as the limbs become increasingly paralysed and the coma deeper. Survival depends entirely on the levels of nursing skill available and death usually takes place around the second year.

The diagnosis is not easy to make in the early stages of the disease and the fundus picture, which is striking, often provides the clue. The posterior pole is a uniform white colour caused by a deposit of fatty material in the ganglion cells of the retina (Plate I). Right in the centre, at the macula, where there are no ganglion cells, the normal pink colour of the choroid is visible; the so-called 'cherry spot'. This appearance is present in the early stages of the disease.

Other genetic defects affect the whole retina and choroid. Albinos, who lack the normal body pigments and who have very fair hair and light-blue or pinkish irises, often have extremely pale fundi. The maculae in this condition often fail to develop properly. A rather similar fundus picture is found in choroideraemia which is also familial and caused by a lack in the formation of the choroidal blood-vessels. In other genetic conditions the macula only in involved. In Best's disease (vitelliform cyst) there are rounded deposits which look like egg-yolk overlying the maculae, and in Stargardt's disease, which is usually seen in adolescents, a pigmentary change gradually appears at the macula. In these conditions there is a large scotoma (gap) in the centre of the field of vision but the peripheral retina is not involved so complete blindness never follows.

All these genetic conditions have a common denominator: the cones of the maculae fail to develop properly and a clear-cut retinal image cannot be formed. This results in nystagmus; a rapid pendular movement of the eyes which constantly 'scan' the visual picture getting more information than they would were they stationary.

Retinoblastoma

Retinoblastoma (glioma) is a malignant condition which affects the retinae of young babies. It has an exceedingly strong (dominant) hereditary tendency. It causes more heartbreak than any other eye disease of children. For here, the issues at stake are not just sight and blindness, but life and death. There is something like one case of retinoblastoma in every 20 000 live births, and it occurs in both eyes in one-third of these cases. Like any other cancer ordinary cells have gone out of control and in this instance the mad cells are those developing from the inner layer of the primitive optic cup. There may be just one islet of growth in one retina or several in both.

Retinoblastoma usually appears around two years but it may be present at birth and sometimes develops as late as six years of age. One eye is usually more affected than the other. Very often it is first discovered by the baby's mother, who notices a white reflection in the pupil when it catches the light (sometimes described as the 'cat's eye' pupil), or it may come to notice by causing a squint.

Untreated, the tumour grows inside the eye and eventually its mass pushes the lens against the cornea and causes a rise of intra-ocular pressure. Eventually the whole globe may be destroyed. Worse is to follow. The tumour extends along the optic nerve and penetrates its coverings, which are continuous with those of the brain. Once extension to the brain occurs death is not far away.

Fortunately the malignant cells of retinoblastoma are very sensitive to radiation and at the present time this is the main method of treatment. If the tumour is seen sufficiently early, before it has reached a diameter of 10 mm, it is treatable by sewing a radioactive plaque onto the sclera overlying the tumour. If it is more extensive the whole eye is irradiated and in cases where the globe is filled with growth the eye is usually removed. In these cases particular care is taken to remove as much of the optic nerve as is possible. Fresh growths or recurrences are not uncommon in the next five or ten years after treatment so these children are examined at regular intervals up to the age of 12. The survivors, and there are many of them, are potential carriers of the condition. In general retinoblastoma patients should not have children; there are exceptions especially when there are no other cases in the pedigree. It is highly important that genetic counselling be obtained in these cases.

93

Blindness and visual handicap: the facts

Retrolental fibroplasia

In the 1940s and 1950s considerable advances were made in the rearing
of premature babies. Many who a decade before would not have had
the slightest hope of survival developed normally with advances in the
techniques of neonate management. But a disturbing number of these
premature infants became blind. And the odd feature was that in the
very clinics, particularly those of North America where the sophisticated methods of rearing prematures were most advanced, had the
highest incidence of blindness. And this was a new form of blindness,
the actual cause of which baffled the experts. The descriptive term of
retrolental fibroplasia or RLF for short referred to the white mass of
connective tissue which appeared behind the transparent lens of the
premature baby. The more premature it was (and infants with a birth-
weight of only 2 lb were now surviving), the more likely they were to
develop RLF, which came on 5-10 weeks after they were removed
from their incubators.

The breakthrough was made by Professor Norman Ashton in London.
He found that the eyes of newly born kittens reared in high concentration of oxygen that had been used in the incubators of the prematures were similar to those of the babies. But why the greater number
of cases in the North American clinics? The American incubators were
leak-proof and maintained a much higher oxygen concentration than
those of their European counterparts. The leaky ones were safer!

Infections

A century ago the most common cause of blindness in the first year of
life was ophthalmia neonatorum, an acute conjunctivitis which has
already been described under that heading (p. 80). Its treatment is
given on p. 81. Toxoplasmosis, which is a common cause of uveitis
in the young, has been dealt with in that section (p. 45). Congenital
syphilis and its lesions of the cornea and of the uveal tract in interstitial
keratitis are described on p. 34 and syphilitic choroiditis on p. 47.
There are in addition retinal changes which are much less commonly
seen. One of these gives an appearance sometimes described as the
'pepper and salt' fundus, as the periphery shows a sprinkling of brown

94

and yellow punctate deposits. Sometimes the optic nerve becomes atrophic too and in these cases there is serious loss of vision.

Infection from intestinal worms in dogs

Many dog owners think that parks and pavements are the ideal places for canine defaecation; there has been much recent controversy about the medical hazards of allowing this. What are the facts? In a letter to *The Times* of 13 June 1980 Professor A. W. Woodruff of the Hospital for Tropical Diseases, London, sets out the risks to children's eyes from infestation by a worm carried in dog faeces, *Toxocara canis*. He writes:

Sir,
I am happy to tell you that my granddaughter, aged 17 months has been able to walk for five months. She and her parents spent the spring holiday with my wife and me and I had for the first time the privilege and pleasure of taking her for a walk in our local park. She managed splendidly the 550 yards to the children's playground but *en route* we had to bypass several specimens of canine faeces and in the playground she was persuaded with difficulty to avoid the sandpit. On the return journey I counted the faecal deposits and found these to number 12, all lying on our direct route. Moreover I had to protect her from the advances of five dogs even though our walk took place between 9.30 and 10.30 a.m. Having delivered her safely to her parents I retraced our footsteps armed with specimen tubes in which I collected samples of soil at intervals of 34 yards. I also took four samples of sand from the sandpit.

Examination in my laboratory of the 16 soil specimens has revealed that four contained toxocaral eggs. The four samples of sand contained none. Perhaps the notice on the railings of the playground "No Dogs" is having good effect and I congratulate the local council for their perspicacity. The condition of the rest of the park however gives cause for concern. I was able during our walk to observe at first hand and, again with difficulty, to overcome the almost irresistible fascination a toddler has in putting into the mouth interesting objects found. The hazard from so doing is obvious and doubtless helps to explain why most — but not all — patients with toxocaral eye and other damage are children. In Britain each year toxocariasis causes damage to, or loss of the sight of, at least 50 eyes.

After the toxocara eggs have been swallowed they hatch in the intestine and the minute larvae burrow through the gut wall, pass into the bloodstream, and spread widely in the body. One of the most favoured sites is the macula area, where the worm forms an inflammatory mass and eventually destroys central vision. Fortunately the condition is usually present in only one eye. A close watch is needed on the Public Health aspects of this condition. Dogs need to have their faeces examined periodically for adult worms which are white, rounded writhing eel-like affairs some 2–3 inches long. If present the animal should be 'wormed' by a qualified veterinary surgeon. Puppies should be treated routinely.

Injuries to babies

During birth the eyes, with the rest of the head, undergo severe compression. Examination of the fundi immediately after birth frequently shows a number of retinal haemorrhages which may spread over large areas of the retinae. However, these usually clear without causing any ill-effects. Another common birth injury, sometimes caused by the application of forceps, is a paralysis of one or both external rectus muscles. This causes a convergent squint present at birth. Again, this usually resolves by the sixth month and if it fails to do so it can often be treated surgically.

The 'battered baby' syndrome was unknown 20 years ago because no-one believed that anyone would deliberately maim or murder a defenceless child. But once pediatricians were alerted to this dreadful crime numerous cases have been reported although few come to court. This is a social rather than a medical problem. The tensions built up by marital disharmony, poverty, physical illness, or personality defects, and a whining whimpering child who was unwanted in the first place create an explosive situation which often ends by an assault on the baby. The head is the target of attack and massive brain haemorrhages may result. These in turn cause retinal haemorrhages not unlike those already described under birth injuries. The optic nerves may also be damaged. Fundus examination of a suspected battered baby often provides the evidence necessary to prove the criminal action and the baby may be saved from further assault and removed to a safe place.

Optic atrophy

Optic atrophy, or death of the optic nerve, is a very common reason for blind registration in children but the precise cause is often never discovered. Optic atrophy is recognized with the ophthalmoscope by the fact that the optic disc, instead of being pink in colour changes to white because the capillaries which nourish it become smaller and finally disappear. However, the disc in children is normally paler than in the adult, and mistakes in diagnosis may be made for that reason.

Optic atrophy and blindness following lesions of the optic nerves, chiasma, and optic tracts are described in the neurology section (p. 78), so all we need deal with here are the reasons for optic atrophy in children. In the absence of firm evidence birth injury is often cited and the verdict in these cases must be 'not proven' unless there is other evidence of brain injury such as mental retardation or nerve paralysis.

Expansion of the fluid spaces in the brain (brain vesicles) with enlargement of the skull occurs in hydrocephalus and may also occur in spina bifida. Further, there are malformations of the base of the skull giving a deformity called oxycephaly (tower-skull). All these conditions are commonly associated with pressure on the nerves and subsequent optic atrophy. Sometimes infections such as meningitis may cause atrophy by causing adhesions in the vicinity of the optic nerves. In some of these cases a limited degree of vision may be retained and in these nystagmus is common. A small proportion is treatable by neurosurgery.

13

Blindness in the Third World

How many blind people are there in the world? The answer is staggering: if you define the blind as those who are so handicapped by their sight that they are limited in the work that they can do the answer would be about 42 million. Most of the blind are to be found in the under-developed countries. At the present time the problem is increasing. Although the birth rate is dropping in the developed countries it is still rising in much of the Third World. The figures speak for themselves. At a recent World Fertility Survey conference it was stated that the United Nations projection predicted that the world's population will be 6000 million in AD 2000, some 50 per cent higher than it was in 1978. The peak is unlikely to be reached until AD 2050 when there will be 11 000 million people on a rather overcrowded planet.

We cannot then look for a reduction in the number of the blind because of any drop in the world population. There is another problem too, and that is that the medical manpower and the financial and administrative resources are likely to be reduced and not increased for the next two generations. In short, more people are going blind than are being cured of blindness and something drastic will have to be done if the trend is to be reversed.

In the Third World, of course, people suffer from the same degenerative eye conditions as they do in the developed countries. Macular degeneration, glaucoma, and diabetic retinopathy are present to the same degree and myopia and cataract more so. But in addition the Third World countries suffer additional blinding diseases caused by poor hygiene, overcrowding, and poverty: infections such as trachoma, onchocerciasis, and leprosy and also deficiency diseases such as vitamin A deficiency and beri-beri. Blindness from all these causes is largely preventable and there is effective treatment for all of them. The problem in the under-developed countries so often is that of getting the patient to the doctor or the doctor to the patient. Cataract is an excellent example of this.

Blindness in the Third World

Cataract

Cataract is found world-wide and there are thought to be 17 million blind from this cause alone. The cataracts do not differ in form from one part of the world to the other but they develop in younger people in India and other hot climates than they do in temperate ones. Treatment requires very efficient organization because of the great numbers of cases which require it and the limited number of surgeons available to carry out the necessary operations.

Dr G. Venkatswamy, of the Madurai Medical College, S. India, gives a vivid account of the organization of cataract camps and the problems inherent in operating on several hundred cataract cases in a single day. Writing in 1971:

At present we are conducting eye camps only in buildings such as schools, colleges, halls, and public buildings. The public within a radius of 20 miles is informed of the date and time which the camp will be open. Publicity is conducted free of charge through the government radio stations. In addition we use newspapers and loudspeakers attached to the van as it passes through the villages. However, in spite of all our efforts, communications are still very poor. The message does not spread easily. The blind person is usually confined to his home, and the information, even if it reaches him, does not always help unless he can find some money and be brought to the camp. In a recent survey in two villages within two miles of the camp, we found that nearly half of the people were unaware of the existence of the camp. Another discouraging factor is that people may think that they are too old for an operation and accept blindness as a part of old age.

Our camps usually start on a Saturday, when we examine all the patients and select the cases for operation. All cases of cataract and immature cataract with visual acuities of less than two metres in the better eye are admitted for surgery provided they have no obvious infection of the lacrymal sac or other external infections. The eyelashes are cut and a sterile pad and bandage is applied. We call this a trial bandage.

Cataract operations are performed on the second day. The patients are awakened early in the morning and the doctors examine their trial bandage. If they show discharge the eye is not operated on but antibiotic ointment is applied and they come to another eye camp at a later date. Those who have no discharge are given breakfast and their eyes are washed and made ready for operation. The medical officers, nurses and other staff are prepared for the operating theatre before 6 a.m.

He goes on to describe the operation which is done under local anaesthesia with mild sedation. Particular care is taken to prevent infection. The operations follow standard techniques but are streamlined where possible as the time allowed for each case is from 5 to 10 minutes; and seven surgeons, working at seven operating tables, may perform 60 or 70 operations in an hour! Their physical stamina must be amazing. After the operation both eyes are bandaged for 24 hours and the patients are fed and nursed by volunteers. At the end of that time the eye is examined by a doctor and any necessary drops are applied. After 7 days the patient is allowed home. Because of the care in pre-operative selection and treatment, and the skill of the surgeons, the complication rate is remarkably low. Finally, at a postoperative visit a 'cataract' (+10.0) lens is supplied and the patient is able to see clearly again.

Trachoma

Apart from styes and lid cysts trachoma is the most common eye disease. Some 500 million people are afflicted and 2 million of these are blind. Trachoma has a very wide geographical distribution, but is mainly found in the Third World countries.

Trachoma is an infection which runs a very prolonged course. It is caused by a chlamydia, which is an organism half way between a bacterium and a virus. It is spread by insects, usually flies, but a body louse will serve. Trachoma is usually contracted at an early age, mostly before the fifth year. Squalor and poverty, dirt, and flies all help to spread the disease. Any marketplace of the Middle or Far East will provide ample opportunity of observing the actual inoculation. Runny-eyed little children unconcerned or oblivious of the flies crawling over their faces and eye-lids do not so much as raise a hand to discourage their dangerous visitors whose previous landing place may well have been a lump of excreta or a sufferer from active trachoma. In fact trachoma often co-exists with a purulent (pus-forming) conjunctivitis contracted at or about the same time.

In the first few weeks after the infection has started the eyes itch and water. The lids are swollen and the conjunctivae are red and thickened. After some weeks these acute symptoms pass away but the chlamydia slowly infiltrates the conjunctival surface of the eyelids, forming

100

characteristic little nodules rather like minute sago grains, which are called lymphoid follicles. Later still, and this may take two or three decades, the tissues become scarred and contracted. This is the final stage and the sufferer is no longer infectious. The lids buckle inwards and the lashes rub the cornea (trichiasis, p. 83) which is already grey and scarred and has lost its transparency due to the invasion of its substance by blood-vessels (trachomatous pannus). The condition goes from bad to worse as the rubbing of the ingrowing lashes causes ulceration of the cornea and further scarring.

If the case is treated in the early stages considerable help may be obtained by the use of local drops of sulphacetamide or by tetracycline ointment. It is more usual, however, to be presented with a case which has progressed to follicle or scar formation. The inturning lashes can be returned to their original position by simple plastic surgical procedures and it is not difficult to train surgical orderlies to do this. Trouble often arises later on when major surgical operations such as removal of cataract or corneal grafting has to be carried out. This sort of operation is much more difficult to do when there is trachomatous pannus present as the corneal vessels start to bleed and obscure the operation field.

The most important treatment for trachoma is undoubtedly preventative. A campaign of instruction of a population at risk will pay dividends. Insistence on measures of hygiene such as personal cleanliness the improving of the water supply, and the adequate covering and disposal of refuse have worked wonders in many areas. 'If the flies go the trachoma goes with them' is a truism. But this is not all. It is always necessary in endemic areas to have periodic population surveys to determine the incidence of the disease, its severity and the age groups principally affected. If for example the main reservoir of infection is in children the whole child population may be most effectively treated by daily treatment with tetracycline ointment carried out for 2 or 3 months in the schools.

Onchocerciasis

Onchocerciasis or 'river blindness' is a parasitic disease which, according to World Health Organization, infects some 20 to 30 million people. Many of these lose the sight in both eyes, albeit very slowly.

Blindness and visual handicap: the facts

One of the most extraordinary features of the condition is that it was unknown to the developed world until just a century ago; and this despite the fact that it must have been afflicting mankind for thousands of years. This is presumably because the main localities where onchocerciasis is rife are isolated rural communities in darkest Africa. In some native villages up to 30 per cent of the inhabitants are infected. Later, across the Atlantic, a second nidus of infestation of onchocerciasis was subsequently brought to light. If you look at a map showing the distribution of 'oncho' (which is less of a mouthful and the name it goes by in ophthalmic parlance) you will see in Africa, that oncho is prevalent in the vast belt of rain forest stretching from the East to the West of the continent and including most of the countries of tropical West Africa, Zaïre, Southern Sudan, Kenya, and Tanzania. The central American countries in which oncho is endemic lie in the same latitude North and South of the Panama canal. Is there some connection between these two areas? Perhaps. The slave traders who wrenched so many Africans from their homes in the Old World to exploit them in the New, used this sea route and they may have brought the oncho with them.

Oncho is a typical parasite in that in its life cycle it lives in more than one host. In this case the main host is man. Its other host is a small

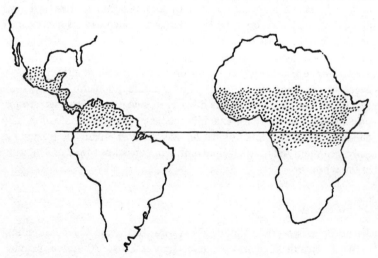

Fig. 7. World distribution of onchoceriasis.

blood-sucking fly and the transference of oncho from man to fly and fly to man goes on unceasingly. The fly has the engaging name of *Simulium damnosum*. It is rather smaller than a common house fly and black in colour. It also has a peculiar hump on its back and for this reason is often called the 'buffalo gnat'. The fly likes to live near fast-running well-oxygenated water so it is often found in the rushing streams of a tropical rainy season or in larger fast-running rock-strewn rivers. It also has the nasty habit of selecting man-made dams and irrigation channels which provide beach-heads of invasion to districts farther downstream. The fly lays its eggs on a stone or plant stem underwater fastened to it by a sticky gelatinous glue. The eggs hatch in 2–3 weeks and fly larvae emerge. These anchor themselves against the stream by means of a sucker and after further growth develop wings and hatch into the adult fly. Off they go then to find a good meal in the blood of a man.

The flies have strong jaws which quickly bite through the skin and this enables the fly to suck blood from its victim, which it does with the greatest ferocity. Now if the man has oncho he will have in his skin numerous little eel-shaped micro-filariae and these the fly draws into its stomach with the blood. The micro-filariae burrow their way through the wall of the stomach and eventually get into the muscles of the fly's thorax where they pass into another larval stage of life. These larvae then work their way to the proboscis of the fly and hope soon for a second victim; as the fly has only a few days of life left to it. Let us suppose that this time the man has so far in his life not contracted oncho. But as the fly bites, the larval filarae invade the wound and a new case of the disease has come into being.

It may be many years before our new case gives any sign of having contracted the disease. In the meantime some of the larvae have developed into adult male and female forms, about an inch or so long. These breed and the breeding sites form nodules under the skin from the size of a pea to that of a walnut. From these nodules millions of microfilariae emerge, not all at once but over many years. They burrow their way in and under the skin and get to most parts of the body but the place where they do the most damage is the eyes for both are usually involved.

The cornea is frequently attacked and the presence of microfilariae sets up a keratitis. Sometimes sectors of the cornea become quite opaque. The iris is also frequently involved and this may set up a secondary cataract or glaucoma. In these cases it is often possible to make out microfilariae swimming freely in the anterior chamber when the eye is examined with the slit lamp. The choroid is also often heavily infiltrated by filariae. The structure which, when involved, causes the most serious effect of all, complete blindness, is the optic nerve.

When a high proportion of the inhabitants of a rural area become blind the economic and social effects are disastrous. In the best of conditions many communities only just manage to exist at near starvation level. If 20 per cent or more of the population cannot do their share of food producing an extra burden is thrown on the rest. The able-bodied leave the village to the blind who then are in a pitiable state living out a kind of twilight sub-life in which they sink more and more deeply into a state of apathy and inertia.

Treatment of onchocerciasis is unsatisfactory. Surgical removal of the nodules especially those on the head is often advocated. This has the effect of removing a reservoir of microfilariae which are constantly being discharged into the skin tissues. Drugs especially those used for combating parasitic worm infections, are not very suitable because although living filaria cause little reaction in the tissues, dead parasites produce poisonous substances which make the patient feel very ill; as so commonly happens in medicine, the treatment is worse than the disease.

A more promising line of attack is to eradicate the fly before it has a chance of biting and thus stopping short its cycle of reproduction. The favourite breeding sites of the fly can be identified by experienced entomologists and these can be sprayed with chemical insecticides in much the same way that malaria-carrying mosquitos are eradicated. At present however these measures are not very efficient and extremely expensive, and as the end results are hard to evaluate they are likely to receive a rather low priority in countries with an already strained medical budget.

Vitamin deficiency

Vitamin deficiencies develop insidiously and occur sporadically in a population at risk. The most important precipitating factors are undernourishment, especially with regard to protein intake, often caused by poverty or famine, occupations involving prolonged physical strain, or debilitating conditions like tuberculosis and measles. Nursing mothers are also at great risk as they deplete their own stores of protein and vitamins giving milk to their babies. Although these conditions are most likely to be found in the Third World it must never be forgotten than vitamin deficiency is by no means uncommon among the elderly poor or alcoholics living on tinned foods in straitened circumstances in the developed world. The eyes can be affected in vitamin A or vitamin B deficiency.

Vitamin A is present in a wide variety of foods especially liver, dairy produce, and green vegetables. The countries in which cases of vitamin A deficiency occur are those of Asia where 100 000 children are blinded each year. There are in addition another 150 000 sufferers in the Middle East, Africa, and South America. These numbers are increasing in line with the global food production which has fallen in the past decade (UN Food and Agriculture Organization).

There are two eye diseases which are caused by vitamin A deficiency, xerophthalmia and keratomalacia. Xeropthalmia is the less severe condition. It causes a dryness of the eyes and the conjunctivae, which, instead of being bright and glistening, lack lustre and look dry. Sometimes deposits of a foamy secretion form on the exposed 'whites' of the eyes; these are called Bitot's spots and quite easily seen with the naked eye. The tear flow is reduced and owing to the lack of mucus the conjunctivae are not properly moist. Later the epithelium of the corneae becomes dry, wrinkled, and gradually opaque with of course severe loss of vision. If seen in the early stages both the corneal and conjunctival lesions can be reversed by treatment. Sometimes the condition causes night blindness. This is associated with multiple white spots at the periphery of the retinae.

Keratomalacia is a far more serious condition which sometimes follows xerophthalmia but may occur independently of it. It is always associated with a grossly defective protein intake. In a matter of days first one and then both corneae become ulcerated and softened and finally melt away so that perforation of the eyeball occurs and without its protective tunic, infection of the interior of the globe rapidly follows and complete blindness results. This tragedy comes about so quickly that all sight is often lost before medical help is obtained. Sometimes one cornea is less affected than the other and in these cases a simple operation in which the cornea is 'buried' temporarily under the conjunctiva may preserve useful vision.

Both in xerophthalmia and in keratomalacia the treatment is by massive vitamin A therapy. This can be given in the form of injection in severe cases or by tablets in others. Under famine conditions it is necessary to screen the population at risk and treat prophylactically where necessary.

Beri-beri is a nutritional disorder found in populations whose diet is deficient in vitamin B. Most cases occur in the Far East where polished rice (that is rice without the husk) is the main food. Chronic diarrhoea, heavy manual labour, and lactation may precipitate the condition.

The main general symptoms are a neuritis which causes painful feet and wasting of muscles (the dry form of beri-beri) or progressive heart failure with oedema (the wet form, also called epidemic dropsy). The eyes may be affected in the wet form and a very insidious form of chronic simple glaucoma develops. Beri-beri responds rapidly to treatment by thiamine.

Leprosy

Most people know something about leprosy, a scourge that has been laid to the back of mankind for thousands of years. The Bible abounds in the lore of leprosy; whole pages of Leviticus are devoted to priestly instructions as to its diagnosis and management. One of the most dramatic stories is the account of the miraculous cure of leprosy given by Elisha to Naaman the Syrian. Naaman, after some demur, was washed pure in the waters of the Jordan and subsequently Elisha's dishonest servant Gehazi to whom the disease was transferred makes his exit from the scene himself a leper.

It is of interest that archaeologists can identify the incidence of leprosy in ancient communities from the evidence left by bones, particularly skulls. There is a very characteristic loss of the four front (incisor) teeth of the upper jaw due to the invasion of the gum-bones by the leprosy bacillus. Furthermore in leprosy the terminal bones of the hands and feet are often missing or stunted.

Leprosy has rightly been feared for the dreadful disease that it is but there are many misconceptions about it; one is its supposedly high rate of infectivity. This is untrue. Leprosy is caused by a micro-organism called myco-bacterium leprae but we will call it by its less scientific name of the leprosy bacillus from now on. One of its unusual character-istics is that it has an extremely slow rate of reproducing itself. Most micro-organisms which cause disease multiply themselves in a matter of minutes or hours (for example the staphylococcus which causes boils and styes) but the leprosy bacillus takes about a fortnight. This means that leprosy develops very slowly and is not the highly contagious dis-ease that was once thought. If for example a husband or wife contracts leprosy there is only a one in twenty chance that their partner will develop the disease.

Most sufferers from leprosy probably get infected in childhood, but show no symptoms until the second or third decade. There is consider-able controversy as to how they contract the infection. Until quite recently it was thought that direct skin-to-skin contact was necessary but it is now felt that the most likely source of infection is from leprosy of the mucus membrane of the nose and conveyed to others by minute droplets in coughing or sneezing. Leprosy is found in conditions of overcrowding, squalor, and poverty wherever it may be. The highest incidence is in the urban ghettos of the great cities of Asia and South America but the kraals of Central Africa and peasant villages of South East Asia also provide the right conditions for the disease to spread.

The WHO has a register of lepers from all countries and on it there are 3.5 million names. These are proven cases who have had or who are still under treatment. However it has been estimated by the WHO Expert Committee on Leprosy that the true global figure must be nearer 12 million. Leprosy is not confined to the tropics and sub-tropics or to the underprivileged countries. In the year 1979 there were 360 lepers in Britain. There is one statistic that apparently has not been worked out and that is the percentage of lepers whose sight is affected. A 'guess-timate' in an editorial in the *British Journal of Ophthalmology* in 1981 gives a figure of between half to three quarters of a million blind or partially sighted lepers in the world.

Blindness and visual handicap: the facts

When the leprosy bacilli get into the body the tissues which are primarily attacked are the peripheral nerves. These are the nerves which radiate from the brain and spinal cord to all parts of the body. They are of two kinds. Motor nerves which supply the muscles of the head, trunk, and limbs and sensory nerves which send sensations of pain, touch, and pressure from the skin and joints to the brain. Once inside the nerves the leprosy bacilli multiply, still very slowly and cause the nerve fibres to thicken and become knobbly so they can be felt as knotted cords under the skin, but at the same time the nerve fibres die. The nerves are attacked in a very haphazard way so that a sufferer may lose the sensation in his right foot and have a paralysis of the muscles of his left forearm. Because of the knobbly thickening of the nerves the condition is called the tuberculoid form (nothing to do with tuberculosis incidentally) and the disease is confined to the peripheral nerves. There is however a much more serious form, lepromatous leprosy, in which the leprosy bacilli get disseminated to all parts of the body including the skin, mucus membrane of the nose, internal organs like the liver, and some of the bones. Among the most serious effects is involvement of the interior of the eye.

The blindness of leprosy is often accompanied by a further deprivation. The loss of the sensation of touch. In the tuberculoid form there may be no sensation in the hands and walking is extremely difficult when there is anaesthesia of the soles of the feet.

The sight is frequently lost in leprosy, both in the tuberculoid and lepromatous forms. In the former this is caused by a paralysis of the lid muscles. This causes an inability to close the eyes properly (lagophthalmos) and as a result the cornea and conjunctiva become exposed and dry especially during sleep. In addition the lashes often become distorted and rub against the cornea which becomes abraded and finally ulcerated (trichiasis). Finally the ulcer may cause perforation of the cornea and infection of the interior of the globe and loss of sight invariably follows.

In the lepromatous form of the disease the bacilli settle in the uveal tract and set up an iritis and choroiditis. The iritis, like other manifestations of leprosy, comes on insidiously with little in the way of warning symptoms like pain or redness. Intra-ocular adhesions often form

108

causing secondary glaucoma. If the inflammation of the choroid affects the central areas of the fundus macular vision will be lost.

The eye complications of leprosy are treated on the same principles as any other disease. A close watch is kept for any drying of the cornea and artificial tears applied every few hours may be sufficient to prevent it. In other cases plastic surgery to the lids to effect lid closure or rectify the position of inturning lashes. Uveitis, choroiditis, and secondary glaucoma are treated exactly as has already been described in the sections dealing with them.

General treatment for leprosy is always needed. The drug most frequently in use at the present time is Dapsone, a sulphone introduced in the 1940s. The great difficulty in treatment is that it has to be kept up for long periods. In the tuberculoid form for at least 3 years and in lepromatous cases for life. All very well for those living within reach of medical support but obviously not a practical proposition for a sufferer living in a remote rural area.

Epilogue

Sir John Wilson writes:

People do not really go blind by the million. They go blind individually, each in his own predicament. In the formulation of strategy and objectives we must keep in view the individual and his community as the reality behind the abstraction of world poverty and disease.

Blinding malnutrition is not an abstraction. It is a blind village girl in Bangladesh — hungry, frightened, frail, utterly weary, with a demanding baby at her breast. Onchocerciasis is not just a disease category. It is a West African village where blind farmers plant grain along a straight piece of bamboo and a hemp rope leads blind women to the well. Cataract surgery is not just a programme. It is an Indian eye camp where, after an operation costing five dollars, an old man looks out on the hills and a child is startled by the first shock of sight . . .

He should know. Sir John is President of the International Agency for the Prevention of Blindness and his book *World blindness and its prevention* should be read by anyone concerned about this problem.

Part II
Living with blindness
ERIC BOULTER

14

Introduction

Blindness is relatively rare in Western cultures, where only about two in every thousand of the population are registered so; but it is difficult to understand why many people feel embarrassed when meeting those who have lost their sight. Occasionally blindness is even equated with loss of intelligence or diminution of one or more of the other senses, particularly hearing. (Most blind people can recount innumerable instances of being addressed in terms that might normally be used for talking with a child − or in a near shout! Blind people must resist the temptation to react by engaging in unnatural behaviour in an attempt to redress the balance!)

Misunderstandings about the nature of blindness often originate because of lack of knowledge concerning the point at which declining sight comes to be recognized as such in medical parlance, legislative provision, or eligibility for supportive services.

The fear of the dark inherent in most young children can leave a lasting impression, and in the minds of many individuals blindness is synonymous with blackness or the complete absence of light. Yet this is not necessarily so, and the attitude of the sighted towards blind people might change if it were more fully understood that blindness can vary widely in degree. Less than one in ten of those officially listed as 'blind' live in a state of complete darkness. The majority remains able to perceive light and even large objects. So blindness may deprive its victims of sight, but not necessarily of light.

Some people are born blind; for others blindness may occur later, either suddenly or gradually. Cases of sudden blindness, for example as the result of an accident, represent only a relatively small proportion of the total number. In most cases blindness is the culmination of a lengthy period of gradual sight loss resulting from the progression of an eye disease such as those described in earlier chapters. So most people who become permanently blind or whose visual loss has been very severe before their eye condition becomes stable may experience months or even years of declining vision. This 'period of grace' should be used to prepare for the day when they may be forced to perform even relatively simple tasks with little or no reliance on vision — and, if wisely used, can serve as a most valuable bridge between the sighted and the non-sighted ways of life.

It is therefore in the best interests of those threatened with blindness that they should become aware of that possibility at the very earliest stage in the treatment of their eye defect. However, the ophthalmologist naturally will remain optimistic for as long as possible concerning the effectiveness of his treatment: it is unnecessary for every person seeking treatment for an eye condition to have dangled before him the spectre of partial or total blindness.

Some ophthalmologists and general practitioners are excessively reluctant to reveal the true facts to their patients, thereby reducing the likelihood of full and effective rehabilitation. They should assist him to take, as soon as possible, the first essential step in the life-rebuilding process — namely acceptance of the fact that, while life may never be quite the same, well-proven measures are readily available which will enable the patient to live in a modified but still thoroughly satisfactory manner.

An equally damaging situation can arise if the patient is unwilling to accept an unwelcome prognosis, and this may often set in motion a lengthy, costly, and in most instances fruitless quest for a 'miracle cure'. There have been countless instances of patients who, at enormous expense, have travelled the length and breadth of their own countries and abroad, grasping at non-existent straws, seeking the 'good news' that is not to be found. Real harm can be caused when the victim closes his mind to the possibility of sustained visual loss and refuses to prepare himself for that eventuality. Unwillingness to recognize that a new way of life has to be evolved will simply impede effective rehabilitation.

However, if all concerned will join with the patient in facing up to the inevitable, preparing for the future with optimistic courage, the results of such endeavour will be wonderfully rewarding.

15

Blindness in the community – a brief historical review

From ancient times blindness, like other handicaps, has been the cause of fear and rejection. Blindness has always been one of the most greatly feared of physical infirmities and it appears that in the earliest cultures the sightless were rarely permitted to live a normal life span or to discharge any contributing role in the family or tribal unit. This attitude changed gradually, with the passage of centuries, as new cultures and civilizations emerged and gained ascendancy, so that fear began to be laced with pity and rejection with a certain level of compassion. Those without sight, while still being debarred from discharging any responsible role within the family or the community, were nevertheless freed from the fear of individual or mass extermination and were permitted, as beggars, to cling to life around the edges of the community in which they existed. Historical records of many different civilizations reveal the presence of blind beggars, indicating that people of the day were willing to give food and other gifts to them and were motivated by pity, compassion, and perhaps by superstition.

In Ancient Greece and Rome, some of the earliest indications of community action are discernible in the allocation to blind beggars of well-chosen locations for the gathering of alms such as the gates of the cities, the steps of the temples, and around civic buildings. And yet many people, including some great leaders, still felt that nothing was gained by keeping blind people alive. At one point the citizens of Rome were exhorted to refrain from giving food and drink to blind beggars, as to do so would be a double evil. First, that which was given would be lost to the donor and, secondly, it would unnecessarily extend the life of misery being endured by the recipient. Plato and Aristotle gave their support to the practice, then current, of putting to death imperfect infants, including those who were blind. In Sparta and Athens, formal rituals were developed for determining whether the degree of imperfection in the young was sufficient to justify their destruction and it was generally ruled that those who were blind should be put to death. There is good evidence, too, that in Rome the practice of ending the lives of physically handicapped babies was prevalent, as records show the sale of small baskets in which blind and infirm infants would be placed prior to being cast into the river Tiber. In Thebes many infants were killed, and those whose lives were spared were frequently sold into slavery.

Yet throughout this early period of history there developed among the populations of many lands a gradual, but clearly perceptible, growth of recognition concerning the innate worth of all human beings and, although many centuries were to pass before the mass of blind people could derive direct benefit from planned services for their education and welfare, they came at least to enjoy the right to life, the receipt of alms, and, in isolated instances, the personal support of influential people.

In China it was recognized that blindness freed the sightless from the distractions of everyday life, enabling their minds to ponder the mysteries of the world. Some gained enviable reputations as soothsayers, being sought out by many in high office. In China, too, music, which was throughout history to be so closely associated with blindness and with the individual lives of blind people, was recognized as being a unique outlet for their talents and early Chinese writings contain references to the blind men who, with songs and gongs, travelled the land bringing enjoyment to their listeners while making their contribution to the growth of public awareness of the abilities that were latent in those without sight. In India blind people began to memorize the stories of past events and to travel the countryside reciting the histories and fables of bygone ages. This cult was also practised in Japan where some blind men came to be welcome guests at the courts of the mighty, where they recited from memory stories and records from the annals of the past.

And so it was that in the Hebraic, Christian, Muslim, Buddhist, and Hindu cultures the place of the blind became more secure. Other than in a few lands where barbarism still prevailed blind people were conceded the right to live. Members of the public became attuned to their responsibility as alms-givers and evidence was gained from the example of some blind people, particularly those of wealthy and privileged background, that even without sight people could have active minds and develop artistic talent through which they could make a marked contribution to the life and culture of the day.

Blindness in the community — a brief historical review

With the spread of Christianity, particularly across Europe, the practice of offering charity to all who were in need, including those with visual and other defects, continued to develop and while few, if any, real efforts were made to provide for the educational training of those without sight, the provision of food and shelter, clothing, and other basic necessities of life became common practice, culminating in Paris in 1254 with the foundation by Louis IX of l'Hôpital des Quinze-Vingts. This was a special residential home for 300 blind people (thus the name — fifteen times twenty) drawn from the streets of Paris and elsewhere in France and staffed by priests. Some effort was made to provide a modicum of instruction and training in simple crafts and a number of blind thinkers of the day, freed from the constant battle for physical survival, added the fruits of their talents to the growing reservoir of positive contributions being made to thought and life in the communities in which they lived. For the most part, however, the residents of the Quinze-Vingts continued their former lives as beggars but with the advantage that they did not have to spend the alms they received on food, shelter, or clothing. L'Hôpital des Quinze-Vingts has continued to be dedicated to the shelter, care, and training of blind people or the cure and prevention of blindness, and is now a hospital for eye patients and a centre for the training of ophthalmologists.

Whilst the purposes for which it was established and the results achieved by the Quinze-Vingts at the time of its establishment were elementary by today's standards, it was outstandingly important in the long history of service to the blind people and the growth of understanding about blindness, being the first recorded case of acceptance by the State of responsibility for the succour and care of visually handicapped people. It was, therefore, the forerunner of many similar enterprises later to develop in Europe and elsewhere, such as residential homes for needy, lonely, or elderly blind people and, in a sense, of the well-equipped rehabilitation centres of to-day with their highly trained staffs of specialists.

Later Paris was to be the setting for yet another step along the long highway towards personal and vocational fulfilment for blind people, for it was there in 1784 that Valentin Hauy established the first school for the formal academic and vocational education of blind children. The story of how Hauy was moved to compassion and pity by the sight

117

of a group of blind beggars performing antics in quaint garb and suffering the derision of passers-by in an attempt to earn alms is well known. He resolved to do something permanently to improve the lot of sightless people in France and elsewhere.

With the founding of his famous school, whose pupils were to include the illustrious Louis Braille, Valentin Hauy launched the modern era of education for blind youngsters and, with it, laid the foundations of all future action for the organized instruction of blind people, leading to today's pattern of widespread accomplishment by the sightless and their integration as fully participating and totally accepted members of their communities. He was one of history's greatest and most successful champions of the blind. The success that he achieved was so striking, his work such a bright star in the firmament, that within the space of a relatively few years the new experiment of providing formal educational opportunities for the blind had taken root throughout Europe and beyond. The impact of Hauy's pioneering work may be gauged by the fact that, between the opening of his Paris school in 1784 and his death in 1822, further schools for the blind had opened in Liverpool (1791), Bristol (1793), Vienna (1804), Berlin and Milan (1807), Amsterdam, Prague, and Stockholm (1808), St. Petersburg and Zurich (1809), Dublin — a Protestant school (1810), Copenhagen (1811), Aberdeen (1812), Dublin — a Catholic school (1815), Brussels (1816), Naples (1818), and Barcelona (1820).

This rapid and widespread development of educational opportunities for the sightless served as the turning-point in the modern history of planned development to meet the special needs of those without sight. From that moment on the blind could themselves serve as co-partners in this process.

Since those days the coalition between seeing and non-seeing for the strengthening of blind welfare, theory and practice, has become ever stronger and the results of such action can be seen in many countries in the steady growth and increasing effectiveness of service activities. The acceptance by blind individuals, and by organizations of blind people, of ever greater responsibility for the planning and administration of those activities which affect their lives has been profoundly welcomed and fostered by all who believe in the ability of the sightless to shape their own destinies.

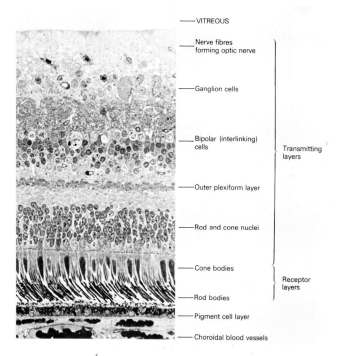

VITREOUS

Nerve fibres
forming optic nerve

Ganglion cells

Bipolar (interlinking)
cells

Transmitting
layers

Outer plexiform layer

Rod and cone nuclei

Cone bodies

Receptor
layers

Rod bodies

Pigment cell layer

Choroidal blood vessels

1. Section of retina magnified 550 times. (*Courtesy of Dr John Marshall.*)

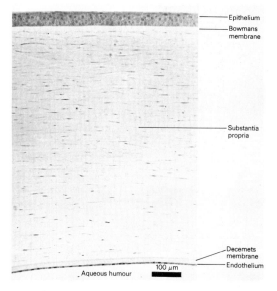

Epithelium

Bowmans
membrane

Substantia
propria

Decemets
membrane

Endothelium

Aqueous humour

100 μm

2. Transverse section of cornea magnified 195 times. (*Courtesy of Dr John Marshall.*)

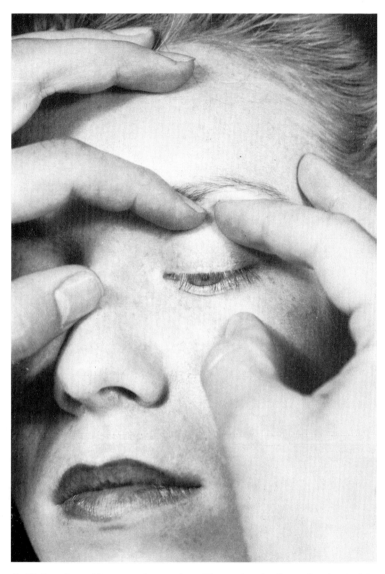

3. Estimation of intra-ocular tension. The patient is directed to look right down. The forefingers are placed on the lid above the tarsal plate. The left forefinger steadies the globe while the right gently palpates. The resistance offered to the palpating finger gives an estimate of the tension.

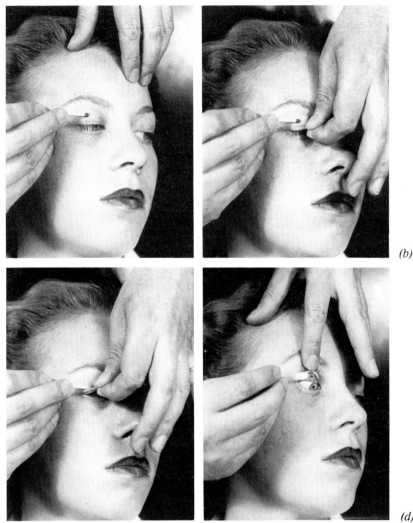

(a)

(b)

(c)

(d)

4. Eversion of the upper lid and removal of sub-tarsal foreign body. (a) The patient must look down and remain looking down throughout the operation. The match is placed just above the upper lid crease which marks the upper border of the tarsal plate. (b) The lid is drawn away from the globe by the lashes. (c) The lid is drawn forward and upwards around the end of the match which is gently depressed at the same time. (d) The foreign body lying in the tarsal sulcus is removed by a cotton-wool stick. (*Photographic Department, St. Bartholomew's Hospital.*)

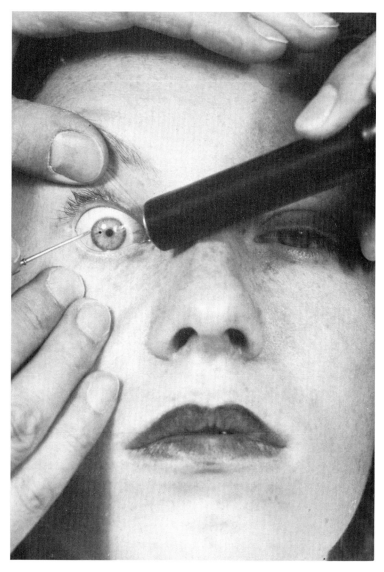

5. Removal of corneal foreign body. The patient is directed to fix the gaze on some distant object. The left thumb retracts the upper lid to prevent closure during the operation. The hand holding the spud or other instrument is steadied by resting the lower three fingers on the patient's cheek.
(*Photographic Department, St. Bartholomew's Hospital.*)

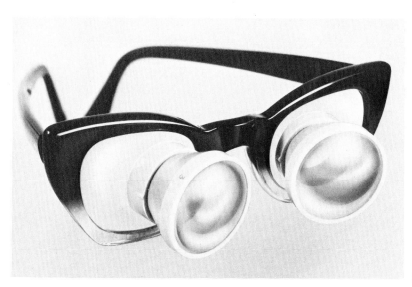

(a)

(b)

6. Low-vision aids: (a) For near: a binocular magnifying device leaving both hands free. (b) For distance: a clip-on telescopic lens with variable focus for occasional viewing, television, theatre, etc.

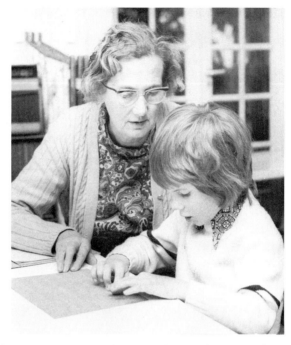

7. A blind youngster at one of the RNIB's Sunshine Houses learns to read braille.

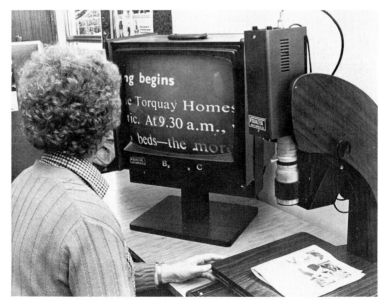

8. Close-circuit television can enable many partially-sighted people to read ordinary print.

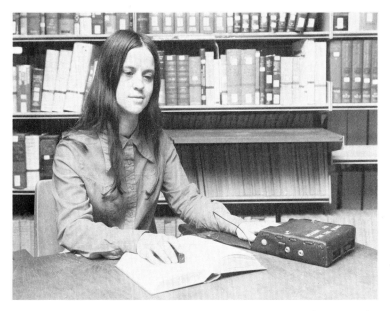

9. The Optacon enables this blind person to read ordinary print by touch.

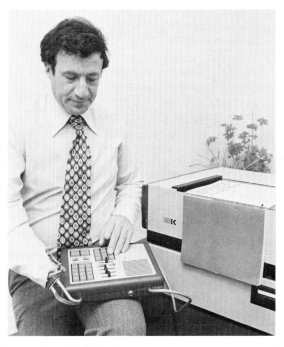

10. The Kurzweil Reading Machine uses synthetic speech to enable a blind person to read ordinary print.

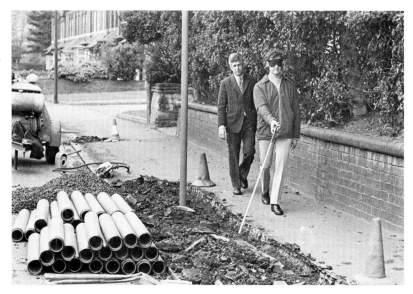

11. With adequate instruction, the long cane technique enables blind people to travel safely even in difficult terrain.

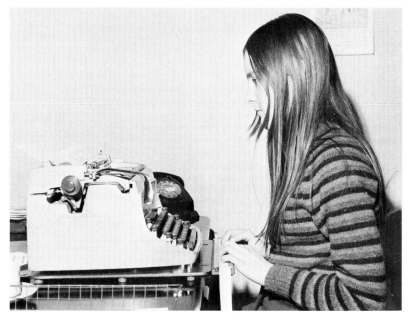

12. This blind shorthand-typist transcribes on to the typewriter material she has recorded in braille on paper tape.

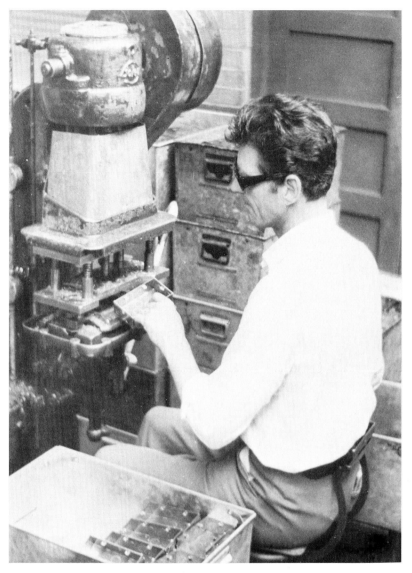

13. A blind factory worker operates a power press.

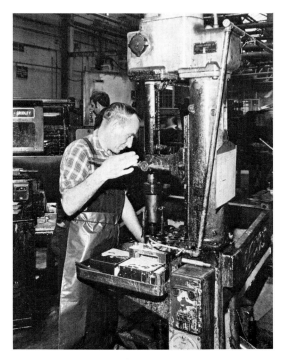

14. Blind workers discharge many important functions in industry. This man is operating a drilling machine.

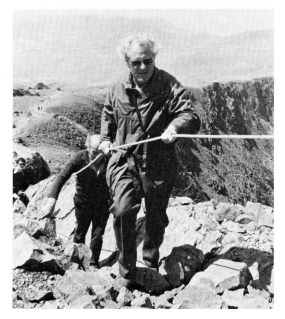

15. Patients from St. Dunstan's undergoing basic rock-climbing training.

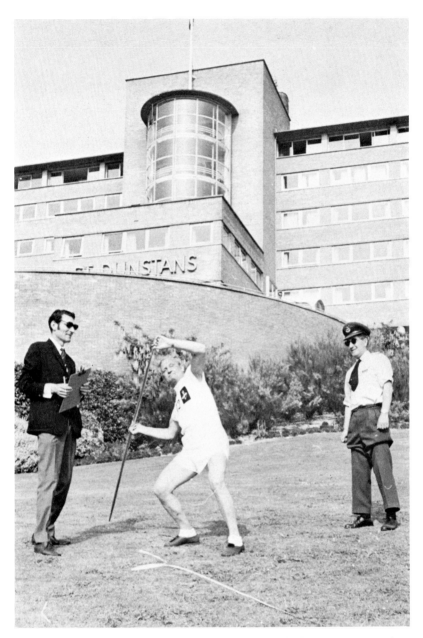

16. Sporting and recreational activities play an increasingly important part in the lives of rehabilitated blind people.

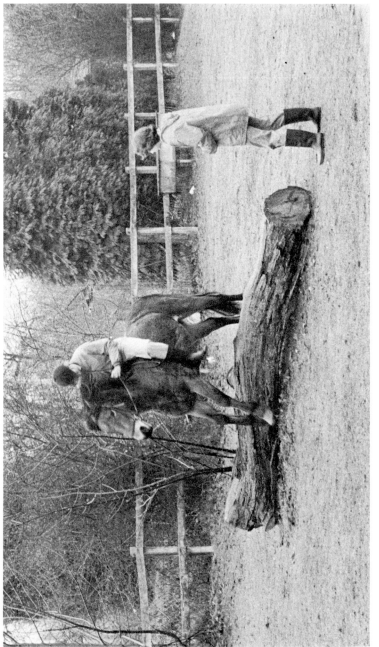

17. Bare-back pony riding helps this blind pupil to develop self-confidence.

16

Movement and travel

Regardless of the age at which blindness occurs, the restrictions it imposes on the power of movement of all kinds are bound to cause frustration. Without conscious thought those who can see are able to judge distances, detect obstacles, recognize danger-spots, and observe traffic movement and the multitude of other factors involved in any pedestrian activity. The newly blind person has to learn to function in an unfamiliar environment, lacking the visual clues upon which he has previously relied: for the first time the environment seems hostile. Problems of mobility can be very real indeed, even within the familiar walls of his own home.

As with most things in life there is for all blind people and those around them a right and a wrong way to proceed. This is particularly true in the areas of mobility and travel and the right ways are best discovered and absorbed through special training. Even when safe movement about the house and relatively comfortable passage in the immediate neighbourhood has been achieved, life patterns will continue to be impaired until the blind person can with relative confidence embark on longer journeys, including the use of public transport: he no longer has the options of riding a bicycle or driving a motor-car.

Unless the difficulties of mobility are overcome true rehabilitation and restoration to a more normal everyday life will not occur. Well-planned mobility training services have evolved in many countries which, together with the use of guide dogs and mobility devices, can immeasurably broaden the travel horizon of visually handicapped people, giving them a new spirit of confidence.

This is a vital element in the total conquest of blindness, for the achievement of ease of travel is the key to participation in many other activities of daily life.

17

Reading, writing, and communication

It is the inability to read and write by normal means that brings home to the newly blinded person, perhaps more than any other factor, his need to rely more than ever before on the help of others. Some blind people live with close family members or intimate friends with whom they are prepared to share every aspect of their lives. But many are not so fortunate and blindness creates for them a situation in which few, if any, aspects of their personal lives can be completely confidential, as the contents of correspondence remain unread until transmitted to them by a third party.

This is also the case with the despatch of private correspondence. Until the blind person is able to achieve the required level of accuracy with typing or to communicate with other blind people by braille, most of his contacts with others, except for those conducted face-to-face or by telephone, will require the participation of another individual. Here again the newly blind person relinquishes privacy.

During the process of rehabilitation, training can be given in a number of methods of communication, including typing, braille notetaking and the use of a tape recorder for maintaining and retaining information on a variety of subjects. Yet the writing difficulties imposed by blindness are never totally eradicated as, for example, the blind person needs help in order to fill in and sign a printed form.

When entering a crowded room the blind person is unable immediately to recognize and approach those individuals with whom he wishes to converse. In a babble of conversation he will find it difficult fully to comprehend remarks which may be addressed to him by his near-neighbours: sighted people rely to a considerable extent on lip reading and the facial expression, gestures, and general demeanour of those with whom they converse.

All people who are blind experience difficulty in keeping in touch with current events. In this respect the radio has an invaluable role. The element of sound in television transmissions is extremely useful to blind listeners but, as this medium of news and entertainment is designed principally in a visual form, it is less satisfactory than radio.

In spite of this, orthodox channels of communication, particularly those in printed form, remain closed to those without sight. This factor can severely prejudice the opportunity for blind people to participate on equal terms with the sighted in many aspects of life, including the educational and vocational spheres. It can, for example, impose additional strain on the sightless in their efforts to maintain normal and natural conversation with those around them. Their exclusion from so many of the usual avenues of information gathering may cause them to feel so ill-informed on details of news and current events that they may become passive listeners rather than active participants.

Of all the forms of physical disability, excluding certain types of mental immaturity, blindness is the most difficult to overcome for the full development and practice of reading, although the skills necessary to overcome the difficulties are relatively easy to acquire. Although very real, the impediments to verbal communication need not be a permanent barrier to participation in educational, vocational, and social fields.

Braille

Whether for study, work, or for recreational or informational purposes, it is important for a visually handicapped person to have access to books and other published materials. Since the invention of Louis Braille's ingenious code, early in the nineteenth century, it has served as one of the most important methods by which blind people read by touch. It is extraordinarily flexible in that it can be used for all languages; for music, mathematical and scientific symbols: for shorthand; and virtually any other purpose for which normal print can be used.

There are now braille printing houses in all the major countries of the world and there is a constant exchange of books and magazines around the globe by organizations and libraries for the blind and between visually handicapped individuals. Such world-wide exchange has been promoted by international organizations of and for the blind, and by the programme maintained by the United Nations Educational, Scientific, and Cultural Organization and the World Council for the Welfare of the Blind since 1950 to encourage uniformity in the application of braille symbols for different languages, for mathematical purposes, and for music notation.

For blind people whose touch sensitivity is not seriously impaired a knowledge of braille can lead to a more or less normal reading pattern, although of course there will always be less material available in braille than in ordinary print. Nevertheless, there is a very considerable quantity of braille material available on loan or for sale and all blind people who feel capable of taking instruction should do so. In most advanced countries courses of instruction can be taken at home, a day centre, a residential rehabilitation centre, or by correspondence course. Learning to write in braille adds substantially to a blind person's self-sufficiency in normal activities of daily life.

The Royal National Institute for the Blind (RNIB) in London and the Scottish Braille Press in Edinburgh are the major printers of mass-produced braille within the United Kingdom and catalogues listing the many titles available from them will be sent on application.

Modern technology in a variety of forms is being utilized by RNIB to achieve maximum output of braille for recreational and instructional purposes. Sophisticated print recognition equipment transfers to digital computer tape the contents of the printed pages of ordinary books, the tapes then being used to motivate automatic machines which convert ordinary print into braille and either emboss the braille symbols on metal printing plates, which are used for mass production of popular publications such as magazines, or produce the braille material directly on to paper when only short runs are required. If the print recognition system does not lend itself to the production of any particular item, the material is typed by key punchers and translated into contracted braille on to digital tape prior to printing by either of the means that have been described. Similar procedures have been adopted for the computerized production of braille music as a result of valuable research at Warwick University. A substantial increase in the number of braille magazines that can be published has been effected through the introduction of an automated production line. Procedures such as these are enabling RNIB to keep pace with the ever increasing demand for braille reaching it from blind people in all parts of the United Kingdom and abroad.

In the United Kingdom the blind reader can also become a member of the National Library for the Blind based in Stockport; the books are sent to and from members by Freepost. The NLB stocks thousands of braille books including many which have been hand-transcribed by the library's corps of paid and voluntary transcribers.

A very wide range of braille periodicals including Weekly News Summaries, is now available, either free or at nominal subscription rates. Catalogues of textbooks, and other material which can be loaned to non-students, are also available. Smaller libraries of braille publications have also been set up by many local societies for the blind.

In the United States the Library of Congress, which is a department of the Federal Government, provides through its National Library Service for the Blind and Physically Handicapped a free braille library service for blind people. Books of all kinds are circulated by mail with free postal privileges by the 56 regional libraries which are maintained in all parts of the country. Most of the books contained in these libraries have been machine printed through contracts between the Library of Congress and certain private agencies for the blind, particularly the American Printing House for the Blind, Louisville, Ky., the National Braille Press, Boston, Mass., and Clovernook Printing House for the Blind, Cincinatti, Ohio. Many volumes are also hand-transcribed by volunteers and to maintain this group of workers at full strength, the Library of Congress offers a braille training course by post. Training is also provided to blind individuals who may wish to prepare for work as braille proof readers. The National Braille Association co-ordinates the work of volunteer transcribing groups and a catalogue listing the publications they have produced in Braille is published by APH. By contracts with private agencies such as American Foundation for the Blind and American Printing House for the Blind, the Library of Congress funds an extensive research programme to improve the quality and quantity of braille material made available to readers throughout the United States, much of which can also be procured on loan by blind readers in other countries if application is made to the Library of Congress by their national organizations for the blind.

Close contact is maintained between the Canadian National Institute for the Blind and the Library of Congress on all matters relating to the production and distribution of braille and other reading media for the blind and a growing quantity of braille is produced by CNIB by computerized and traditional publishing methods as well as through the activities of volunteer transcribing groups. Some reading matter for the blind can be secured at Public Libraries but a direct mail service is also maintained from CNIB Headquarters and its provincial branches. Similar services are maintained by the several State-wide institutes for the blind in Australia, by the Royal New Zealand Foundation for the Blind and the South African Library for the Blind.

Moon type

For blind people whose touch sensitivity is limited, instruction may be given in the use of Moon type (raised type) as an alternative reading medium although this system is used in only a few English-speaking countries. At present, despite continuing research, there is no effective method of writing in Moon type. All Moon production is undertaken by the Moon Branch of the RNIB which can provide a list of the publications available including books, reference works, and periodicals. The NLB and many local libraries also contain titles in Moon type. However, the demand for embossed books in this form is relatively small when compared to braille and the number of titles available is limited.

Talking Books

Many older people who become blind lack the ability or the inclination to learn to read by touch and, equally, many people who are acquainted with the braille or Moon systems occasionally enjoy being read to rather than expending effort and energy in deciphering embossed type.

The value of Talking Books to blind people of all ages is reflected in the extensive programme that is maintained by the National Library Service for the Blind and Physically Handicapped in the United States, fully funded by the Federal Government to provide a free reading service for the visually impaired. Books on all subjects representing a cross section of the titles available at public libraries are circulated free of postal charges by the 56 regional libraries maintained under this programme. Books are recorded on 4-track tape cassettes and on 33, 16, or 8 r.p.m. micro groove discs and play-back machines for each of these recording methods are provided to blind readers on free loan. The Library of Congress Talking Books are recorded under contract by the American Foundation for the Blind and the American Printing House for the Blind, each of which also undertakes research programmes for the improvement of the service. Volunteer groups in all States provide substantial additional material for the regional libraries, State organizations for the blind and visually handicapped individuals, the national co-ordination of such activities being the responsibility of Recording for the Blind Inc. Many popular magazines, including *Reader's Digest* are now being produced in recorded form and information about sources and subscriptions can be secured from the Library of Congress or any of the State agencies for the blind.

Well over half the registered blind people in the United Kingdom are members of the British Talking Book Service for the Blind. Close to 4000 titles have been recorded and are loaned to members of the library who are provided with play-back machines and regularly updated catalogues. This service is subsidized by the RNIB and many local authorities or local voluntary societies for the blind are prepared to pay or help with the membership fee.

UK Talking Books are recorded on magnetic tape on special long-playing cassettes with up to 12 hours' playing time. The cassettes can be used only on the specially designed Talking Book machines which are maintained by service volunteers. The cassettes are sent to and from the library by Freepost.

The Canadian National Institute for the Blind maintains an extensive Talking Book programme based on the use of the 4-track tape machine used in the United States by the Library of Congress. Many of these books are recorded by professional readers at CNIB's Toronto Studios but, as in other countries, a considerable number are recorded by volunteers working in their own homes. This service is free to blind readers, being supported by Government grants and the cassettes are sent by Freepost from CNIB national or provincial headquarters or in some Provinces are available from Public Libraries. The New Zealand Foundation for the Blind, which offers a direct mail Talking Book service for blind readers in that country, has opted for the British system which uses a cassette with 12 hours' playing time using 6-tracks for reading purposes and 2-tracks to provide an indexing facility. This system is also used in South Africa and some of the States of Australia, although in both countries alternative systems are also in use making it necessary for interested individuals to direct their enquiries to the State or local organization for the blind.

Sadly, many blind people are forced to lead sheltered and often solitary lives and, among the whole range of blind welfare services, the Talking Book is perhaps the most important in terms of the number of hours of interest, enjoyment, relaxation, and instruction that it can bring.

Talking Newspapers

Enforced isolation often makes it extremely difficult for blind people to keep in touch with current events and local affairs, and recently there has been a rapid growth in the publication of Talking Newspapers and Talking Magazines, frequently organized by groups of volunteers. Talking Newspapers consist of items recorded on tape drawn from the columns of national and local newspapers, frequently supplemented by items of special interest to blind readers. Talking Newspapers are usually recorded on standard compact cassettes for an ordinary commercial tape recorder. A growing number of magazines is also now available.

Recorded textbooks

Recorded textbooks and other material required by visually handicapped people attending universities, polytechnics, and other levels of Higher and Further education are also available through leading agencies for the blind. Well in advance of the start of each academic year the student must secure from his department head or tutor a list of the required reading for that year and indicate those books which are most urgently required. Much of the recording for this service is undertaken by volunteer readers working in their homes, each being familiar with the subject matter that he is recording; professional readers also work in some of the programmes for example at Britain's Student Tape Library, particularly on material required by blind students of the Open University, the course outlines which are often issued at very short notice. The Student Tape Library is also equipped with high-speed equipment to make copies of books which have already been recorded. In addition, the library has several thousand recordings made in earlier years which

126

may be drawn on by accredited students. All the services of the Student Tape Library are free to registered visually handicapped persons.

With support and help from the Library of Congress and often under the aegis of Recording for the Blind Inc. volunteer recordists are at work in their homes throughout the United States reading onto tape the textbooks that are required by blind people at all levels of education and particularly those pursuing university and college studies. This is a free service and students may obtain their books in cassette form from regional libraries for the blind or direct from members of the recording group concerned. In most States the Department of Education or the Department of Special Education makes similar provision for the production of recorded textbooks particularly for blind pupils attending public school classes and a number of local private agencies for the blind offer similar help. In a number of other countries, including Canada, Australia, New Zealand, and South Africa, the organizations responsible for the operation of Talking Book programmes referred to earlier in this chapter are equally involved in the provision of recorded textbooks for students sometimes producing the books in their own recording studios but more frequently by the recruitment of volunteers and the co-ordination of their work.

Radio

Radio enables the blind to remain well informed about current events, and many years ago the British Wireless for the Blind Fund was created to ensure a set would be provided to any blind person in need in the United Kingdom. Special programmes are designed and carefully compiled to meet the needs and wishes of blind people. The pioneer programme, 'In touch', is transmitted weekly by BBC Radio 4. It is presented by a team of talented visually handicapped presenters and each programme includes items of interest to blind and partially sighted listeners throughout the country. The guests who appear on the programme, many of whom are themselves visually handicapped, provide information about new developments, special events, tips for overcoming some of the problems of blindness, and items of general interest. A Quarterly Bulletin containing brief summaries of the programme is issued by the BBC and a publication, also entitled 'In Touch', is a valuable reference resource. Many local BBC and independent radio stations also transmit special programmes for blind listeners.

The United States has made more dramatic progress than any other country in the provision of special radio programmes for blind listeners. Many local radio stations now transmit for several hours each day programmes of special interest and entertainment geared to the needs of the visually handicapped. These programmes are carried on special FM wavelengths and serve a vital ingredient in the pursuit of instruction, gathering of information, and the enjoyment of leisure by those without sight. In areas where these special programmes do not yet exist, most US local radio stations have adopted the same pattern that exists in Britain, Canada, and Australasia by transmitting weekly programmes containing items of interest and guidance for the visually impaired.

18

Access to services

There has been built up in all advanced countries and many of the developing lands a range of services covering the needs of blind people of all ages designed to hasten adjustment, provide education, rehabilitation, and training, enhance employment prospects, improve financial circumstances, and extend welfare provisions for those without sight. Such programmes may be provided by governments or other statutory bodies or by private voluntary organizations, but more commonly through a combination of both. The general pattern of such services is very similar in each country but the method of gaining access to their benefits and the relationship between national, provincial, and local governments and voluntary societies is not constant. Equally, it will be recognized that there are inevitable differences in terminology and varying emphasis on certain aspects of the total service. For instance, in the United Kingdom the level of visual acuity at which a person is recognized to be blind within the accepted meaning of that term is expressed in metres, whereas in the United States, Canada, and some other countries the measurement is given in feet. Almost everywhere eligibility for help from organized programmes is achieved by inclusion in a Register of Blind or Partially Sighted Persons but responsibility for the compilation and maintenance of such registers is not constant. In the United Kingdom each local authority maintains registers for the area it administers but annually supplies statistical information to the Department of Health and Social Security for inclusion in a National Return. In the United States, the information is maintained at State level, the administration normally being handled by State Commissions for the Blind. In Australia, too, State governments have a statutory responsibility but much of the detailed work is performed by voluntary agencies. In Canada and New Zealand a high level of responsibility is discharged by national voluntary societies and their regional offices. Almost everywhere national legislative provisions describe in general terms the financial and service programmes that must be maintained to alleviate the problems of blind people, yet within any given country the methods that have been introduced to implement the law at the state, provincial, or local level may differ sharply. This is particularly true with respect to the extent to which voluntary organizations participate in the development or provision of services.

In this volume it is not possible fully to describe all the forms of assistance that may be available to those who have suffered severe visual loss in each of the countries to which we make reference, nor to list the requirements for inclusion in a register of blind or partially sighted persons. As a general guide we discuss in this chapter the steps that are taken in the United Kingdom to identify blind and partially sighted people and thus set in motion the statutory and voluntary services that can be utilized to achieve improved living patterns for those without sight. In other chapters, and in the Appendix to this volume, we give information about many of the governmental and voluntary organizations in other countries which can provide more precise information on all aspects of service to the blind.

Registration

In the United Kingdom access to the benefits of many of the services for the blind depends on inclusion in a Register of Blind Persons or a Register of Partially Sighted Persons. These registers are maintained by each of the local authorities throughout the country and are the responsibility of the Social Services Departments in England and Wales and the Social Work Departments in Scotland. These Departments are charged statutorily with responsibility for offering a wide range of services for blind people, either by themselves or through the activities of voluntary societies which act as the agents of the local authorities.

Registration is not compulsory and the consent of the individual must be secured before action can be taken. We would very strongly recommend, however, that the necessary steps to seek registration be taken to ensure that all available help will be offered. Usually full advice will be given to the patient by the ophthalmologist who is treating his or her eye condition. But in some instances loss of sight may be irreversible and gradual and the patient may have ceased regularly to consult a specialist ophthalmologist. The visually handicapped person or, with

130

his consent, a close relative or friend should then approach the Social Services Department of his local authority, requesting that an investigation be undertaken to determine whether he qualifies for registration as a blind or partially sighted person. In each case a Consultant Ophthalmologist must complete a form and forward it to the Director of Social Services of the local authority concerned. In the case of a baby or young child the staff of the local education authority should take the necessary steps to secure registration if the visual defect is sufficiently serious, or alternatively the parents should ensure that the Social Services Department institutes investigatory action.

The local authority concerned will then arrange for a qualified social worker to visit the home of the affected person to explain the range of local and national services that are available and how to ensure that he receives the benefits of any of the available services which could be advantageous.

There are three categories of registration, each of which is designed to ensure that the patient qualifies to receive the most appropriate form of assistance:

(1) technically blind;

(2) partially sighted;

(3) partially sighted people who are entitled to use the services appropriate to those who are blind.

The consultant ophthalmologist must indicate to which of the registers he considers his patient should be admitted. Registration in one of these categories is not necessarily permanent and, should the vision of the registered person improve or decline, he can be re-examined by a consultant ophthalmologist. If necessary the patient will then be re-classified or removed from the register altogether.

The legal definition of technical blindness appears somewhat imprecise but has been found, in practice, to serve as a very satisfactory base. It requires 'that a person should be so blind as to be unable to perform any work for which eyesight is essential'. It should be noted that the word 'work' does not necessarily apply solely to paid employment but also to the normal tasks of daily life. Thus, for example, a child at school, a non-working housewife, or a retired individual would not be excluded simply because they were not in paid employment. The consultant ophthalmologist indicates the level of visual acuity in each eye, as generally accepted levels of visual acuity give the criteria for registration in one of the three categories.

The category 'technically blind' includes patients who can see with the better eye 3 metres or less that which a person with normal vision can see at 60 metres. It is recognized, however, that even though the patient's central vision may be within the parameters described, the effectiveness of his sight may well be complicated by defects of peripheral vision. Therefore, should peripheral sight be seriously impaired he may still be registered as technically blind if he can see at up to 6 metres what can be discerned at 60 metres by a person with normal vision.

There is no statutory definition for the classification of partial sight but any individual who is substantially and permanently handicapped by defective vision is normally eligible for the welfare services extended by local authorities and some central government departments. The consultant ophthalmologist has to provide certain additional information to indicate whether in his judgment blindness is likely to occur at an early date, and whether the nature of the visual defect is such that the patient could benefit from the provision of training for employment or for the other appropriate services. This is very important for those partially sighted people with an unfavourable prognosis for the retention of a reasonable level of vision. In such cases the local authorities may ensure that, while some useful vision is retained, the patient can take a course of rehabilitation which will enable him or her to acquire the techniques of daily living which will be so essential at a later stage. It may even enable him or her to be prepared for and placed in a job which can be performed satisfactorily without the use of sight.

We would like to reiterate that for most people who are technically blind or partially sighted, inclusion in the appropriate register is the first essential step towards the benefits of the welfare services – statutory and voluntary, local and national – that may assist them substantially to overcome their handicap and to resume a rewarding and purposeful way of life.

Local goverment

The staff of each local authority should include a number of persons who are specially trained to provide helpful assistance to the blind and partially sighted persons in their case-load. Following an initial visit from a social worker to establish the general condition, financial status, and basic requirements of the registrant, a staff member known as a Technical Officer for the Blind will be assigned to each case. This officer's job is to assist the visually handicapped person to overcome many of the problems imposed by blindness. The manner in which this is accomplished is individually tailored to each blind person. He or she will regularly visit the blind person in his or her own home and will ensure that the special techniques are acquired which will enable a visually handicapped individual, except when prevented by serious additional infirmity or extreme age, to overcome the problems of normal living. Arrangements may be made for regular home visits to provide guidance and help in cooking, cleaning, the care and laundering of clothing, dressing, shaving, applying cosmetics, storing and labelling foodstuffs and other belongings, as well as minimizing hazards and inculcating the client in the skill of free and safe movement within the household. The client should also be helped to venture outside the home with a reasonable level of confidence.

At this point a further local authority staff member known as a Mobility Officer may be assigned to the case, although in some local authorities the responsibilities of the Technical Officer and the Mobility Officer are combined. The Mobility Officer should help the client to start moving about easily first in the immediate neighbourhood of the home and then further afield. The development of mobility skills broadens the client's horizons so that he can undertake shopping expeditions, visits to neighbours, attend church, or join in or resume social activities. The officer who is providing mobility instruction will help with the selection of appropriate travel aids: for example, embossed maps, a long cane, a short stick, or a guide dog. He can arrange for the client to spend a period of residential instruction in the handling and care of a guide dog at a guide dog training centre. It should be pointed out, however, that for a variety of reasons the use of dogs is suitable for only a small percentage of the blind population, and it should not be assumed that the acquisition of a trained dog necessarily provides the solution to all mobility problems.

The Technical Officer should also be qualified to provide braille or Moon instruction (see p. 121) in the client's home if necessary. These and other skills can also be acquired during a short course of residential social rehabilitation at one of the centres maintained by the Royal National Institute for the Blind (RNIB). While some local authorities accept full responsibility for payment of the subsidized training fee some others require the blind client to contribute all or part of the cost.

In some areas the acquisition of social rehabilitation skills can take place at classes at day centres and arrangements can ususally be made for the regular transport of the visually handicapped to and from the centre. Similarly, many local authorities organize recreational activities for those who have sight problems such as clubs at which they can meet other blind people, and use the facilities to pursue interests such as music and drama.

In the United Kingdom Technical Officers of the Blind can give advice on how to gain membership of the National Braille Library and obtain Moon literature, periodicals and newspapers, and Talking Books.

The life-style of the newly blind person can thus be substantially enhanced if the local authority is brought into the picture. For instance, many local bus and underground systems offer free travel or concessionary fares for registered blind people; television licence fees can be reduced; and admission to certain museums and other cultural events may be offered at concessionary rates.

Central government

Responsibility for providing services to meet the needs of blind people in the United Kingdom rests to a considerable extent on local Social Services Departments and local educational authorities. It is, nevertheless, the responsibility of central government departments and, more especially, the Department of Health and Social Security and the Department of Education and Science, to ensure that appropriate standards are maintained. Furthermore, other benefits which are of the utmost importance to blind people are extended as a result of direct action by central government departments. Financial assistance is available to those who are registered as blind persons and this, even though it is considered by many to be inadequate, can reduce the financial strain at the onset of blindness. Despite the difficulties blind people face in travelling even short distances, they are not eligible under existing

134

legislation to benefit from the Mobility Allowance unless they also suffer from other physical or medical disabilities which make it impossible for them to walk. Similarly, blindness unless complicated by very serious additional factors does not permit its victim to qualify for receipt of the Constant Attendance Allowance.

There are two programmes of financial benefit available to registered blind persons. All blind persons (or the blind spouses of sighted taxpayers if a joint return is submitted) are entitled to a special income tax allowance in recognition of the fact that blindness imposes additional living costs. However, this concession does not apply to those who receive non-taxable Government pensions for blindness as a result of war injury or service-related causes. Registered blind persons whose total income is so low that they qualify for Supplementary Benefit from the Social Security Department are entitled to receive a higher rate of benefit than is paid to those who are not so registered. Both of these financial benefits are available only to those whose names are included in the Register of Blind Persons, and not to those on the Register of Partially Sighted Persons.

With the exception of the above financial provisions, the most important services made available to blind people as a result of direct action by government departments relate to the rehabilitation and training of visually handicapped persons who are adjudged to be suitable for employment, and the programme for their placement in appropriate occupations. Both of these services are maintained by the Manpower Services Commission which a visually handicapped person may approach directly or be referred by his Social Services Department.

A blind person's Resettlement Officer or Disablement Resettlement Officer having been assigned to the case, the Training Services Division of the Manpower Services Commission is responsible for ensuring that rehabilitation programmes are made available for those blind people who wish to secure and it is considered likely will be able to obtain employment of a type that could be satisfactorily performed despite the visual handicap. The TSD does not operate its own rehabilitation centres but arranges for applicants to be admitted for residential instruction at the centre maintained in Torquay by the RNIB or that in Ceres, Fife, maintained by the Society for Education and Teaching of the Blind (Edinburgh and South-East Scotland).

Blindness and visual handicap: the facts

In a later chapter we shall describe some of the philosophies underlying the rehabilitation process. Although participation in a formal residential course of rehabilitation probably provides the best preparation for a suitable job and a fuller life, many people make a completely satisfactory transition without attending such a course, if instruction has been given to them by their Technical and Mobility Officers in braille, typing, mobility, personal adjustment, and general skills of daily life.

Once the necessary basic skills have been acquired, the visually handicapped person may undergo a course of formal training for a specific form of employment. The courses available are discussed in Chapter 21 on employment and finance (pp. 162-9).

A blind Person's Resettlement Officer is an official of the Manpower Services Commission and is responsible solely for the provison of services to persons who are visually handicapped. A Disablement Resettlement Officer performs precisely the same function but carries a mixed case-load, working on behalf of people who may be disabled in a variety of ways. If it is felt that the visually handicapped person will be better served by seeking employment either under sheltered conditions or by working in his own home the BPRO or DRO will refer him to an appropriate sheltered workshop where training may be arranged prior to employment in one of the trades practised therein. Potential home workers may be referred for training to one of the several organizations (frequently Workshops for the Blind) which operate home-workers schemes, for example the RNIB which maintains an extensive scheme covering London and the South-Eastern Counties of England.

The Manpower Services Commission, in addition to meeting the cost of residential training or rehabilitation, pays a maintenance grant and issues travel vouchers to enable the client to maintain contact with his home and family. Should such a client subsequently decide to accept a post in a place other than that of his normal residence, he may qualify for a grant to cover or contribute towards removal and resettlement costs. Under the Technical Aids to Employment Scheme items of technical equipment can be provided which will enable a visually handicapped person to perform a function which would otherwise be beyond his powers. Several such items have already been listed as recognized aids for blind workers and others are added from time to time.

Access to services

Braille letters and other braille printed material, Talking Books from and to the British Talking Book Service for the Blind, cassettes to and from recognized Talking Newspapers, and many frequently used items of special equipment can be mailed by Freepost. However, individuals' correspondence by means of cassette recordings must be paid for at the normal postage rates.

As a result of concessions granted by HM Customs and Excise, under the terms of a UNESCO agreement, certain items of apparatus and equipment for the blind enter the United Kingdon free of customs duty. Many such items which are imported by RNIB and other organizations can therefore be sold to blind individuals at lower costs than would otherwise be possible. If a blind individual wishes to obtain from abroad an item of equipment specially produced for use by blind people guidance about the procedure to be followed can be obtained from the RNIB.

19

Blind children

Infants

When parents first hear the tragic news that their child is or will become blind they may experience overwhelming feelings of inadequacy and despair, and as much experienced help, guidance, and support as possible should be made available to them as quickly as possible. Regrettably this does not always occur and, even in these latter decades of the twentieth century, it is not unknown for parents to be left to cope unaided with the problems of the early care and training of blind babies and pre-school-age children. Nevertheless many such parents seek and procure the necessary help even when information about the services available has not been given to them by the doctor, hospital, or child care or social service officers, but others may feel that if their child's blindness cannot be corrected very little of purpose can be accomplished during the years of babyhood and that they must manage as best they can until the question of formal education arises, when most of them realize that some special arrangements will have to be made. In cases such as these the blind child may pass through the critical pre-school formative years in the sole care of young, bewildered, and inexperienced parents who may be overflowing with love but have little or no knowledge about the best way of caring for him. Normal feelings of maternal or paternal love may be overwhelmed by the pity they feel for their tiny blind offspring.

In the days immediately after the birth of a blind child the crushing blow of learning about the physical imperfection of the child may provoke rejection of the infant, complicated by self-doubts. The parents may secretly wonder whether their child has been born blind as an act of retribution for past failings on their part, or they may find that their love for their baby is tempered by resentment at the prospect of a lifetime of burdensome responsibility for a child who will never be able to fend for himself. Happily such reactions are usually short-lived and are normally overcome without medical intervention: the understanding

138

help and support of friends and loved ones is usually sufficient to restore equilibrium to their relationship with the child. In some extreme cases, however, the grief of the parents may be so deep-seated and hold such harmful implications for the future that they are advised to seek psychiatric help.

Children should from their earliest days begin the process of observing, studying, and exploring the world immediately about them; for the normal child this is accomplished in the greatest measure through the use of sight and sound. When a baby sees or hears something, his normal reaction is to reach for it in order to touch it and make further investigations. The blind infant is at a serious disadvantage as he is forced to function without one of the two basic stimuli that motivate the actions and the mental growth of young children. Babies who can see rapidly gain confidence and a feeling of security establishing their orientation to the world around them and automatically detecting any change in it. The blind child should be provided with greater opportunities for personal exploration and physical contact, even at the risk of suffering an occasional minor setback. This may not be recognized by the over-protective parent, who is anxious to shield the child from harm or danger, and blind children are sometimes confined to a cot or playpen well beyond the age when sighted youngsters would have graduated to a world of wider experience.

It is easy for the caring but misguided parent to assume that whilst the baby is in his cot he can come to no physical harm, and to believe that in such manner his well-being is being catered for. But the child should be encouraged to crawl and climb about as the spirit moves him, to touch and learn the size, shape, and density of anything upon which his hands may alight. There will be an occasional tumble and tears but these will be far outweighed by the advantages of the more normal life he is leading and the understanding that physical contact with the people and things around him will engender.

As we have already learnt, blindness does not necessarily mean total lack of vision, and many babies and young children possess a degree of sight which, although greatly restricted, is of inestimable value in the development of their interests, skills, and personalities. As is true throughout life, maximum advantage should be taken of any remaining sight and this fact should be borne in mind when parents are selecting toys and other playthings for their visually handicapped infant. All children gain stimulation through colour and if the visual defect of a blind baby is of a type that has not involved loss of colour sense, efforts should be made to surround him with bright objects of conflicting colour. Equally, things that sparkle and glisten will attract his attention and excite his interest and encourage movement and tactual investigation; but perhaps most of all it is important to provide opportunities for the development of personal relationships both with his parents and with other children. Some parents fear that a blind toddler may suffer physical hurt or rejection if he is allowed to play with other children. In fact, this socialization provides the best opportunity for sowing early the seeds of the establishment of human relationships and acceptance by the blind child, as well as the seeing children who play with him, of the fact that he is a valuable member of a community. Thus the participation of a blind child in playschool or kindergarten activities should be encouraged and persevered with, even if things do not seem to go too smoothly at the outset.

Thankfully, the number of babies who are born blind is declining and the help available to their parents is greater and more accessible than was the case a number of decades ago. Nevertheless, other complicating factors have become more prevalent in recent times, particularly the increased frequency with which blindness in young children is accompanied by other physical or mental defects. Any such combination of handicaps inevitably makes the early care and training more difficult to accomplish.

Parents often wonder whether to choose a kindergarten designed and staffed specifically to meet the needs of blind youngsters, or one in which their blind toddler might derive benefit from the company of children who can see. No generalization can be made in answer to questions such as this, particularly where the early preparation of multiple handicapped children is concerned. Generally speaking the ultimate goal in the rehabilitation of blind and otherwise handicapped people is to help them prepare for the maximum achievable level of integration in the normal community, and the sooner a move can be made to that end the better.

If the multiple resources now available within the community and from many professional and voluntary organizations are harnessed in a co-ordinated way, the prospects for the future happiness, purposefulness, and usefulness of the infants concerned even those in whom blindness is accompanied by grave additional physical and mental defects, are much improved. A number of avenues of help are now available to the parents of blind children and to the visually handicapped child which, if properly utilized and backed up by positive parental attitudes, can go a long way towards minimizing the restrictive effects of blindness. The handicapped child will be able to gain personal confidence, expand his activities and experience and enjoy a reasonably normal childhood with others of his own age group, achieve a level of education comparable with them, and prepare himself for future life as a blind person living in the sighted world.

Nurseries

All children can benefit considerably from attending nursery schools and playschools where, in addition to learning to control their thought processes and develop mental and physical co-ordination, they can gain stimulation from becoming part of a small community. This is equally true of children with a visual handicap; indeed, their need for stimulation of this type may be greater. It is recommended, therefore, that parents of blind children should, in co-operation with their Education Authority, peripatetic teacher, or education adviser concerned, explore the possibility of sending their child to a suitable local playschool. The specialist teacher or adviser will also be pleased to advise the staff of the school about any special provisions that may need to be made to ensure that the child will be able from the outset to participate as much as possible in the school activities. This professional contact will be maintained while the visually impaired child is at the school and this experience can serve as a valuable preparation for more formal education.

There are certain circumstances in which the specialist teacher or RNIB adviser may recommend admission to a nursery school specially designed for the early training of visually handicapped children. In the United Kingdom these nursery schools are known as Sunshine Houses and four are maintained by RNIB. In the United States and elsewhere nursery departments are frequently contained within State-recognized schools for the blind. They are all residential establishments so that children admitted to them must inevitably be away from their families for lengthy periods during the year. Nevertheless, every effort is made to maintain family links to the full, and parents and other relatives are encouraged to pay frequent visits to the Home, while resident pupils are encouraged and assisted to return to their families for weekends and longer holidays. With the increase in the number of visually handicapped children attending ordinary day nurseries, the special residential kindergartens are now more frequently used by visually handicapped children with additional disabilities, physical, mental, or social and the staffs of these programmes have considerable experience in the care and management of such children.

Parents making the important decision about which form of nursery education might be most beneficial should do so only when they have derived as much benefit as possible from consultation with the peripatetic teacher or education adviser concerned. They should also visit the various establishments under consideration to find out more about the routines and resources and to establish personal relationships with the staff members who will be responsible for the care and training of their child.

Education

Important responsibilities rest with the parents of visually handicapped children proceeding either from day or residential nursery schools to primary education, or the parents of children whose sight becomes impaired when they are already attending school. Professional advice should be secured from the educational authority who may consider convening assessment teams, social workers, and others once it has been established that the child is educationally blind. Parents must be aware of all of the possible alternatives so that their final decision is reached as a result of their full evaluation of professional advice from all the relevant organizations and individuals. Usually the choice will lie between a special school for the blind or the partially sighted and a normal day school. The number of visually handicapped children is relatively small and as a result there are only a few special schools each usually meeting a State-wide or regional need.

Many parents are attracted by the possibility of sending their child to a local school so that he can continue to enjoy all the benefits of

142

home life and remain a member of the local community. The theoretical advantages are most persuasive, but a note of caution should be injected because of the very wide disparity between education authorities in some countries concerning the level of supportive assistance that they are able or willing to offer to those day schools to which blind or visually handicapped pupils may be admitted. In many cases blind children attending normal day schools are able to keep pace with their sighted classmates and enter fully into the general life of the school, as a result of the special training given to their teachers, the provision of special equipment, the availability of braille or large-print books, and in some instances low visual aids. However there have been cases where blind children have been encouraged to attend local day schools where few such provisions have been made. A visually handicapped child pursuing his schooling in conditions such as these is doubly disadvantaged. Unless parents can satisfy themselves that adequate supportive provision will be extended to the day school of their choice, they should probably opt for admission to a special school for the visually handicapped.

In all countries of the developed world it is now accepted that blind children, and those with partial sight whose residual vision is seriously impaired, enjoy the same entitlement to education at all levels as is available to non-handicapped children, in that it should be provided at public expense. To implement this philosophy it is also recognized that special schools and programmes shall be provided, that training arrangements shall exist for the preparation of specialized teachers, that educational equipment and books for the visually impaired shall be readily available and that the programmes must be sufficiently flexible to meet the particular needs of blind individuals. There is a growing trend in a number of countries towards the pattern of integrated education through which blind youngsters attend local schools with their sighted friends while continuing to live in their own homes. This pattern of education which was originally pioneered in the United States has since been introduced to a lesser or greater extent by educational authorities throughout the world. A number of factors are crucial to the success of the integrated method of instruction. First, the selection of the children must be undertaken with the greatest care so that those who are mentally, emotionally, or physically unable to compete with other children

143

of their own age group will not be forced into a situation of undue stress. Secondly, there must be full assurance that the child concerned will receive full support from parents and siblings, that the local school in which he is to be integrated has on its staff teachers who have received training in the special techniques of educating those with visual handicaps, or which receive regular and frequent visits from teachers who are so trained. Thirdly, that within the classroom the blind pupil will have readily available in braille, large print or sometimes recorded form all the lesson material and textbooks that are being used by his sighted fellows as well as tape recorders, braille slates, arithmetic slates, and other special devices which will enable him to keep pace. In some places, and particularly in larger schools which have an enrolment of several blind pupils, a special room (sometimes called the braille class) has been set aside for the use of visually handicapped pupils to which they can withdraw for certain periods each day to receive instruction in the use of apparatus, collect brailled or recorded material, and receive special help with educational problems resulting from their blindness. The braille class is supervised by a trained teacher of the blind who maintains contact with other members of the staff ensuring that all necessary lesson material will be available in braille or recorded form at the appropriate time. Where the number of enrolled blind pupils is insufficient to justify the creation of a braille class the functions of the supervisor are undertaken by an itinerant teacher who will discharge the same tasks at a number of schools.

Despite the growth in the pattern of integrated education, it must be recognized that this form of instruction is not suitable for all visually handicapped children and that in many places the factors crucial to the success of the scheme are not yet present. Furthermore, it is increasingly true that blindness in children of school age is accompanied by either physical or emotional difficulties which may preclude the possibility of satisfactory levels of attainment by the child in an integrated setting. Special schools for the blind therefore exist in all countries and will continue to make a major contribution to the development of well-rounded and informed individuals who, upon leaving school, will be ready to assume a responsible place in society. In some of the larger cities children can continue to live at home attending a special day school for the blind, usually being transported to and from school

144

under an arrangement made by the local education authorities. More usually, however, schools for the blind are residential in nature, the children returning to their homes at weekends or during half-term or longer school holidays. Because of the growth in the incidence of dual or multiple disabilities, such special schools must be staffed by teachers who are capable of helping children with a range of additional problems which may include deafness, mental retardation, physical disabilities, emotional disturbance, orthopaedic handicaps, or social inadequacy. Wherever such residential facilities are maintained for blind or partially sighted children, strenuous efforts are made to ensure that the establishment will not become a totally segregated community and the visually handicapped pupils are encouraged and assisted within the limitations imposed by their physical and mental handicaps to participate in a broad range of activities with their fully able counterparts at local schools and in the general life of the city or town around them. Most schools are equipped with special apparatus and aids designed to minimize the effects of blindness and accompanying handicaps. Libraries of braille, large print, and recorded books are extensive and adapted equipment for sport, games, recreation, and leisure pursuits are at hand.

As was stated at the beginning of this section, the cost of providing special educational facilities for the visually handicapped, either through their integration in the normal school system or their attendance at special day or residential schools, is met from public funds. There is, however, no worldwide formula governing the conduct of these educational services some of which are maintained in their entirety by State or local government bodies while others function under the auspices of accredited voluntary organizations with government education departments exercising a supervisory function and a degree of budgetary control. Furthermore, the methods of discharging educational responsibility to blind children, and particularly those who may be categorized as special cases, vary from place to place. For example, in the United States most schools for the blind provide a comprehensive range of educational services from the age of four through High School, separate departments in those schools meeting the special needs of children who are both deaf and blind and those with other disabilities which necessitate very special treatment. The same pattern is observed in Canada, New Zealand, South Africa, and some of the Australian states but the

Blindness and visual handicap: the facts

Royal New South Wales Institute for Deaf and Blind Children maintains a separate school for those of its blind pupils whose visual infirmity is complicated by additional physical or emotional problems. This is equally true in Great Britain where the Royal National Institute for the Blind maintains two schools for blind children with additional handicaps, one at the primary and one at the secondary level. The RNIB also has separate grammar (High) schools for blind boys and girls who display outstanding academic abilities. This is in contrast to the co-educational pattern that exists in most educational programmes for blind children in Great Britain and elsewhere and plans exist for the ultimate merger of the two schools which it is recognized would be advantageous in a number of directions.

In the United States the administration of all programmes for the education of the visually handicapped rests with the education departments or departments of public instruction and are supported by State and Federal funding. In discharging these responsibilities the State Education Departments are responsible for implementing all Federal laws relating to the education of blind children, ensuring that each individual is placed in the most appropriate form of education, i.e. residential or day school for the visually handicapped or integrated into a suitable public school and administering the latter programmes in collaboration with the relevant public schools system. They are also responsible for the co-ordination within their respective States of all programmes maintained on behalf of the visually handicapped children and of their families at the pre-school level and serve as clearing houses for the distribution of braille and recorded textbooks, special educational equipment and supplies required for the further education in all its forms of visually impaired children. While most state schools for the blind are operated directly by State Education Departments, there are a number of special schools which are maintained by private organizations, particularly for the education of those whose visual impairment is complicated by grave additional handicaps. These private bodies are accredited by the State Education Departments which provide financial subsidies. The Federal Department of Education (Office of Civil Rights) administers a law prohibiting discrimination against qualified handicapped individuals in federally-assisted educational programmes while the Office of Special Education administers the Education of the

Handicapped Act and allocate funds to universities and teacher training colleges for the conduct of special training programmes for teachers of the blind and other personnel.

In the United Kingdom the Central government discharges its overall responsibility for the maintenance of educational standards within all schools' programmes for the blind through the Department of Education and Science but local education authorities arrange for the placement of individual pupils in the schools for blind or partially sighted children which meet regional needs throughout the country and for administering programmes under which blind pupils attend local schools. Some schools for the visually handicapped are run by local authorities while others operate within the programmes of voluntary agencies but in all instances the local education authority meets the cost or pays any fees that may be imposed. Nevertheless, all those schools which are maintained by voluntary bodies are subsidized in part by the organization concerned which is authorized to raise money from the public for that purpose. This procedure is followed by some of the regional primary schools, by RNIB in respect of its schools for additionally handicapped blind children and its two grammar schools and by the Royal National College for the Blind which operates a school at secondary and prevocational level with considerable emphasis being laid on instruction with a vocational objective. Special schools for partially sighted children are also located regionally, being operated in some instances by local education authorities and in others by voluntary agencies with the local education authority accepting responsibility either for maintaining the school or meeting fees in respect of children drawn from their own areas.

The Canadian education system for blind children is very similar to that prevailing in the United States with special residential schools existing at a number of places admitting children from their own and neighbouring Provinces. Maintenance of national educational standards for the visually handicapped is the responsibility of the Federal Government but day-to-day administration of the schools and the expanding programmes of integrated education rests with the provincial government authorities which fund all approved programmes. Likewise, in Australia the Commonwealth Government maintains supervision but the delivery of educational services for visually impaired children is a

State responsibility, the programmes usually being operated by private bodies which receive grants from the Commonwealth and State Governments. Within the total programme offered by the Royal Victorian Institute for the Blind, a considerable emphasis is placed on integrated education, more than half the visually handicapped children it serves now attending local schools. The important children's centre and school at Burwood concentrates to a considerable extent on its impressive programme for the education of additionally handicapped blind people including the deaf-blind. It is also the distribution point for the circulation of braille and recorded literature and other educational supplies for those blind children who attend public school. A feature of the programme offered at the New South Wales Institute for Deaf and Blind Children, which also serves a considerable number of those with dual or multiple disabilities, is that the children reside in small units or flats under the guidance of house mothers to create a family atmosphere and stimulate preparation for independent living. A similar approach is in evidence at Homai College near Auckland which school for blind children, including a deaf-blind unit, is maintained by the Royal New Zealand Foundation for the Blind which receives grants from central Government and the payment of fees from those State governments whose pupils attend the college. Partnership between the government and the voluntary sector serves as the basis of South Africa's educational programmes for blind children maintained at eleven residential schools. Here, too, the increased enrolment of multihandicapped children is reported and there are four special units for those with the dual handicap of blindness and deafness.

In recent decades there has been a massive increase in the number of blind people proceeding to university and other levels of advanced education. Whereas in earlier years most of those who were academically able to aspire to become undergraduates selected Law, the Church, or Social Sciences, there is now virtually no Faculty that remains closed to visually handicapped students. In Great Britain, the United States, and all the other advanced countries of the English speaking world, well planned support programmes are available for blind men and women pursuing courses of higher education. With the assistance of State Education Departments, State Commissions for the blind throughout the United States extend financial and tangible support particularly in the provision of equipment and textbooks in recorded, braille, or large-print form. Textbook programmes are also maintained by the Library of Congress, National Braille Association, and Recording for the Blind Inc. In the United Kingdom the required braille and recorded material is principally obtained from the student braille and tape libraries of the Royal National Institute for the Blind while the same organization makes financial grants for the purchase of necessary equipment and to provide personal readers for those books which are not available in any other form. Grants to cover tuition and residential costs are made by the student's own local authority. Similar interaction between Government Departments and national and provincial organizations for the blind prevails in Canada, Australia, New Zealand, and South Africa to support the activities of blind students engaging in studies at all levels of higher education in those countries.

20

Rehabilitation and training

Blindness can strike at any age, but occurs more commonly in those who have already established careers and life-styles and, even more often, in the elderly.

Many people of working age lose their sight each year, and programmes of rehabilitation and training have been developed for their benefit as well as to assist those who may not wish to take up an occupation but who nevertheless seek restoration to a situation of personal independence.

The psychological impact of becoming blind may be profound and frequently results in a total loss of self-confidence. Most vocational and daily living skills are affected and many may have to be re-learnt. New methods of moving safely from place to place have to be acquired, as do skills for reading, writing, and general communication. New techniques have to be adopted by the newly blind housewife if she is to continue to discharge her normal function in life, and sporting, cultural, and recreational interests and activities will need to be reviewed.

The first steps towards rehabilitation are often provided within the home. Yet relatives of those who become blind, while motivated by the kindest of intentions, may become over-protective and impede the progress of a blind person in his efforts to become self-reliant and less dependent on the sympathetic help of others. Therefore it is frequently beneficial for a newly blind person to undergo a course of rehabilitation away from his or her normal surroundings. This possibility should be seriously considered by any person who becomes blind and wishes to remain active, regardless of age. When such rehabilitation courses are undertaken with others who have recently passed through the same experience of sight loss, many of the feelings of embarrassment and selfconsciousness which so frequently accompany the onset of blindness are removed, thus allowing the individual's personality to re-assert itself, and freeing his mind to accept the need for personal re-orientation. The mere fact of tackling new and unfamiliar tasks in a group rather than alone usually has great therapeutic value.

Social rehabilitation

The blind person advised by his social worker, technical or rehabilitation counsellor may decide that a course of residential social rehabilitation should be undertaken. This form of rehabilitation is particularly designed for blind people who are not seeking paid employment and wherever such courses are located, the aim of the operating authority is always to provide a level of trained counselling and instruction designed to satisfy the most pressing needs of each individual, rather than to work to a set curriculum into which all residents must fit.

As most of those seeking courses in social rehabilitation are beyond normal working age and are likely to spend a considerable part of their future life in the home, emphasis is laid on the acquisition of new techniques to meet the requirements of daily life in the family setting. Learning to cook, clean a house, sew by hand or machine, store and identify foodstuffs, select, mend, and launder clothing and linen, set the table, polish cultery, sweep floors, and vacuum carpets all may find a place within the individualized courses. Personal management, including new methods of cutting and handling food on the plate, selecting and applying make-up, shaving without using a mirror, and the multitude of other small but important facets of everyday life can be approached with confidence when the right methods are learnt. Instruction is also provided in free and safe movement within the home and in the street by specially trained Mobility Instructors.

The ability to read and write may be re-acquired through braille or the Moon system. Help will also be given in the retention of handwriting skills using special equipment, and if the client wishes, instruction can also be given in typewriting.

Those undergoing courses of social rehabilitation are also able to learn a number of handicrafts which can provide many hours of enjoyment and interest and, in some instances, be used to supplement the family income. It is not all work and no play during the rehabilitation period, for clients are encouraged to participate in dancing, music appreciation, discussion groups, theatre-going, fishing, walking, and table games. All these form part of the preparation for a well-rounded life in the home environment and contribute to the restoration of personal independence.

In some places the necessary help in adjustment is offered to blind people in their own homes by trained social workers, technical officers, or rehabilitation teachers. Their efforts can be supplemented by the attendance of the clients at day centres which may serve the blind exclusively or have a mixed enrolment of people with varying disabilities. We feel, however, that many more than are at present being served could derive greater and more permanent benefit from residential instruction, even though it may at the outset be difficult to persuade the visually impaired person to leave home. Those directly concerned in Britain should discuss the matter fully with their local authority representatives; and the question of the payment of fees should also be raised. Some local authorities pay in full, but in other areas the blind client is required to make a contribution.

In the United States and Australia enquiries should be made to the appropriate State agency or Commission for the blind. In Canada, New Zealand, and South Africa such approaches can be made to the Canadian National Institute for the Blind, the Royal New Zealand Foundation for the Blind and South African National Council for the Blind, respectively.

Vocational rehabilitation

People who are in employment or who are of working age when blindness strikes should undergo a special course of general and vocational rehabilitation which may lead either to their satisfactory resettlement in their former occupation or open up fresh prospects of satisfactory employment elsewhere. These courses are designed to bridge the gap between the old and new ways of life and in so doing to bring out the qualities of adaptability that are latent within all of us. The newly blinded client should be informed about available formal courses of rehabilitation as quickly as possible following the onset of the disability.

Many of the areas covered during a course of general and vocational rehabilitation are similar to those contained in the social rehabilitation curriculum, being concerned with the performance of common tasks of daily life through the development of new skills and the increased utilization of the remaining senses. But since the final objective in the resettlement of the rehabilitants will be their acceptance or resumption of employment, greater emphasis is placed on certain aspects, such as various forms of hand-work, which are undertaken not simply because of their intrinsic value in the lives of blind people, but to assist the centre's counsellors to judge the manual dexterity and possible vocational inclinations of the clients. More vocationally orientated forms of instruction in such tasks as woodwork, assembly, inspection, turret lathe, and other engineering machine operation are provided and a number of clients proceed to advanced training prior to placement. Braille, typewriting, and other communication skills are specially emphasized and frequently lead on to employment in administrative or commercial posts. Great emphasis is placed on mobility training, as it is pointless to prepare a client for a job if he lacks the ability to travel easily to and from work.

As a result of the work undertaken at the rehabilitation centre and the encouragement that is given to clients to join actively in the life of the town, many blind individuals who have entered the centre with trepidation and doubt have left it imbued with renewed confidence and hope, knowing that the necessary adjustment has been made, that they are possessed of new and valuable skills, and that specialized placement services will be available. In Britain the client seeking vocational rehabilitation will be referred to the Manpower Service Commission by his local authority or he may directly approach the Royal National Institute for the Blind.

In the United States and Australia enquiries should be made to the appropriate State agency or Commission for the blind. In Canada, New Zealand, and South Africa such approaches can be made to the Canadian National Institute for the Blind, the Royal New Zealand Foundation for the Blind and South African National Council for the Blind, respectively.

Training

Whether emerging from a residential rehabilitation centre, completing the process of re-adjustment at home or a day centre, or leaving school, it will be necessary for many blind people to undergo a course of special training to prepare them for employment in the career of their choice. In most advanced countries such training services are available free to blind men and women under existing legislation for the handicapped, being provided in some places directly by governmental agencies and in others by private bodies, voluntary organizations, and employers who serve for this purpose as the agents of the national or State governments. Based on the proven ability of blind workers to excel in certain areas of employment training programmes are now widely available covering a range of professional, technical, administrative, clerical, and manual skills. As a result, the length of the training courses vary considerably.

During recent years increased numbers of blind men and women have successfully completed courses of training as computer programmers and data analysts prior to taking up employment in such occupations, and this field continues to expand as more items of equipment are devised which enable sightless individuals to insert into or retrieve from computers information which can be transmitted in braille or synthetic speech. In most countries training courses in the practice of physiotherapy are available for suitable blind candidates although it should be noted that the practice of this profession by blind people has not been approved by the State health departments in most parts of the United States. In some countries courses in salesmanship can be arranged for those whose bent is in that direction, while in the commercial and clerical fields there is a long and respected history of training opportunities for shorthand and audio-typists (now including word-processing equipment and telephone switchboard operating, including familiarization with boards using speech output).

Either by admission to special training centres or by paid 'on the job' training, blind people can become skilled operators of engineering equipment such as centre and turret lathes, power, punch, and fly presses, as well as skilled inspectors and viewers utilizing highly sensitive devices specially produced for use by those without sight, which can be read with accuracy by touch or through synthetic speech output. Special emphasis should be laid on the possibility of securing 'on the job' training for a wide range of industrial processes under the tutelage of experienced training officers, and when this factor is taken into account the employment opportunities that are opened up to blind people in general industry are almost endless.

For some blind people, particularly those whose visual handicap is complicated by other disabling conditions, sheltered employment in one form or another will continue to be the most appropriate career objective. In almost every country provisions exist for new employees to be trained at the expense of the statutory authority prior to their acceptance as paid employees of special workshops for the blind, many of which are now highly industrialized. Similarly, those who wish to prepare themselves as skilled craftsmen working at home can undergo training courses to that end.

The passport for entry into one of the many fascinating professional and technical careers to which blind men and women may now aspire will be the satisfactory conclusion of a degree or diploma course at a university, college, technical school, or institution of further education. Entry to such programmes of advanced instruction is now freely available to mature students as well as to those in the younger age-group. And in all advanced countries special provisions exist for the admission of blind students within national and local programmes for which financial provision is made by those departments of central or local government which are responsible for educational or vocational rehabilitation services. It is important to note that in all lands blind people pursue such avenues of higher education on a fully integrated basis, joining the student bodies of ordinary colleges in company with their physically able compatriots and thereby extending their experience of serving as respected participants in the life of the communities in which they find themselves.

Guide dogs

Historical records stretching back for well over a thousand years contain innumerable references to blind individuals who have been led by dogs and so enabled to move with greater ease from place to place. And it is equally true that over the centuries many have gained particular solace after the onset of blindness from the unique companionship that so frequently develops between man and dog. However, little more than half a century has passed since the inception of an organized guide dog movement with the animals being bred and trained for the specific purpose of serving as a living travel aid for those who cannot see coupled with the provision of instruction to blind people in the most effective methods of handling their dog guides. In that time the guide dog movement has become worldwide and while it must be stressed that ownership of a guide dog will not for everyone automatically eliminate all the difficulties that accompany the onset of blindness, it can for many provide a means of personal mobility and freedom of action which cannot be secured by other means. In countries where guide dog agencies exist a blind person who is physically able, except for blindness, and anxious to extend his travel horizons can discuss the possibility of guide dog ownership with his social worker, rehabilitation counsellor, technical officer or mobility officer who will be able to advise whether the acquisition of a dog would seem to provide the most effective means of meeting the travel objectives of the individual concerned. If so, detailed advice will be offered as to the steps that should be taken.

In the Western world all guide dog agencies are private voluntary organizations generally raising their income by securing donations from the general public and other charitable bodies but in a few cases charging a subsidized fee to the recipient of a trained dog. Each of the agencies maintains breeding kennels or selects suitable puppies bred elsewhere and conducts the training that will enable them to become the safe guiding eyes for a blind person even in places where crowded pavements and complicated traffic patterns could create profound difficulty. This process begins with puppy walking before the real training of more mature animals is commenced and it has generally been found that bitches prove to be the more capable guides. No single breed of dog is recognized as being most reliable but those in most common use are labradors, golden retrievers, alsatians, and collies, though a number of other breeds and cross-breeds are used in some programmes. When the training of the dog has been completed comes the crucial step of giving initial instruction to the potential new owner and bringing the two together for a course of combined training which is designed to achieve a blend of temperaments which will permit the two to work contentedly together as a unit. At the conclusion of the residential training course, the blind client and his dog are usually accompanied to their home by an officer of the training school which normally provides an after-care service, sometimes providing or helping to secure financial support for the construction of a dog run, arranging refresher courses if necessary, and providing replacement dogs.

In most countries legislation exists by national statute or local ordinance for the protection of guide dog owners including the remission of dog licences and permitting to blind people with trained and properly harnessed guide dogs access to public buildings, hotels, restaurants, trains, buses and other forms of public conveyance, usually on production of some proof that the animal is a trained guide dog. The training agencies in most countries issue owners with an appropriately worded identity card for production on such occasions. In Canada registration with the Canadian National Institute for the Blind is accepted as sufficient proof. Although travel within any country of guide dog and owner is usually assured, it must be noted that some difficulties can arise when international travel is involved. This is occasioned by a stringent anti-rabies legislation in force in some places and particularly island states. In the United Kingdom, for example, guide dogs are not exempted from quarantine regulations and will, on arrival in the country, be placed in quarantine for six months. In most countries, however, the production of a valid anti-rabies inoculation certificate is sufficient to gain entry.

Following valuable experimental work undertaken in Switzerland and in Germany the guide dog for the blind movement was introduced in the United States by the foundation in 1929 of Seeing Eye Inc which continues to provide an extensive service from its headquarters at Morristown, New Jersey but schools are now also maintained by agencies in a number of places including Leader Dogs for the Blind, Rochester, Michigan; Guide Dogs for the Blind Inc, San Rafael, California; Guide Dogs Foundation for the Blind Inc, Forest Hills, New York; Pilot Dogs, Colombus, Ohio and International Guiding Eyes Inc, Burbank, California, which claims to offer a worldwide service.

In Britain the guide dog programme was introduced with the help of an American woman enthusiast who had witnessed the creation of such services in Switzerland and the United States. The impetus that she and others brought to this effort led to the creation in 1931 of the Guide Dogs for the Blind Association. This organization to which potential guide dog owners may be referred by their local authority or approached directly has its headquarters at Windsor, Berks but breeding programmes and the four-week courses for owners with their new dogs are conducted at five modern centres located strategically throughout the country. The Royal Guide Dog Associations of Australia, Kew, Victoria, administer programmes for breeding and training dogs and instructing owners. In addition to its guide dog work this organization also provides general rehabilitation training and instruction in other modes of mobility. Some other guide dog facilities have come into recent operation and those seeking fuller information should approach their State Institutes for the Blind. Similar action should be taken in South Africa where a significant breeding, rearing, and training programme is maintained by South African Guide Dogs Association for the Blind in Johannesburg. A growing number of blind people in Canada have selected the guide dog as the best means of achieving personal mobility and many secure their training at guide dog centres in the United States. Full information about all available services can be secured from Canadian National Institute for the Blind in Toronto or any of its provincial offices. Those in New Zealand who may wish to explore the possibility of securing training prior to becoming guide dog owners should contact the Royal New Zealand Foundation for the Blind in Auckland.

Government and voluntary services

In the United States the administration of rehabilitation and training services for the visually handicapped such as have been described is undertaken by the governments of all States, the relevant departments being known variously as State Rehabilitation Services for the Blind, State Commissions for the Blind, or State Offices of Vocational Rehabilitation. These programmes are funded jointly by the State and Federal governments, the Rehabilitation Services Administration in Washington DC also discharging a national leadership function for the maintenance of standards and the provision of technical guidance for the most effective prosecution of the joint Federal-State rehabilitation programmes. In some instances both at State and local levels federally-supported programmes of rehabilitation and training for visually handicapped people are conducted by accredited private non-profit agencies.

Rehabilitation and training

Close partnership between governmental and voluntary organizations similarly exists in the conduct of rehabilitation and training programmes for the blind in most other Western countries. In the United Kingdom many of the services necessary to achieve readjustment are provided in the home by social welfare, technical or mobility officers of the local Authorities of the areas in which the clients reside. These basic services are frequently supplemented by additional programmes which are conducted by local voluntary societies. Formal courses of social rehabilitation may be undertaken at the special centre maintained by RNIB after referral of cases by the responsible local authorities which may cover the total cost or, in some cases, require the blind rehabilitant to make a contribution. Vocational and general rehabilitation is provided at residential centres maintained by RNIB in England and the Society for Education and Teaching of the Blind (Edinburgh and South-East Scotland) in Scotland, these courses being largely funded by the Manpower Services Commission which also offers training courses in certain vocations for blind people at a skill centre as well as making financial provision in respect of approved training courses elsewhere, including 'on the job' training on the premises of a potential employer. Central government resources are also available for the maintenance of certain vocational courses, such as piano repair and tuning, offered to blind people by the Royal National College for the Blind.

Co-operation between government departments, federal and provincial, and the Canadian National Institute for the Blind, provides the basis for the operation of rehabilitation and training services for blind people throughout Canada. Serving as the agent for the federal and provincial governments CNIB offers instruction and training at its provincial centres and the A. V. Weir National Training Centre in Toronto, all such activities being planned in collaboration with the government's job creation programme. These courses include adjustment to blindness, orientation and mobility, secretarial courses, including word processing, pre-university and middle management training courses and preparation for a number of industrial and manual occupations including retailing, particularly in the management of vending stands and catering facilities.

Extensive and varied programmes for the adjustment, rehabilitation, and vocational training of blind people exist in all the States of Australia

159

and are maintained through close co-operation between Commonwealth and State governments and the several State-wide voluntary organizations such as the Royal Victorian Institute for the Blind and the Royal New South Wales Institute for the Deaf and Blind. Joint planning for the country as a whole occurs at meetings of the Australian National Council for the Blind which brings together representatives of the voluntary organizations which exist in each State and representatives of appropriate government departments. As in most other countries the rehabilitation programmes in the States of Australia embrace personal adjustment, braille and other communication skills, mobility training, familiarization with technical aids and equipment including the Optacon and Kursweil reading machines, vocational counselling and development, and handicrafts, particularly at the rural out-stations maintained in some States. Training is provided for a number of occupations prior to placement in commerce, industry, or sheltered workshops. At some workshops the more traditional trades are being superseded by engineering, packaging, and assembly and many forms of sub-contract work undertaken on behalf of industry.

Programmes of rehabilitation and pre-placement training maintained in New Zealand through collaboration between government departments and the Royal New Zealand Foundation for the Blind follow a similar pattern to that existing in other advanced countries with many of those who complete training at RNZFBs provincial branches or National headquarters in Auckland securing suitable jobs in the open employment market being assisted by a National placement service. Any special equipment required to enable a blind person to undertake suitable work is provided through joint funding by government and RNZFB, including closed circuit television for registered blind persons who retain some sight.

Much of the work undertaken by the South African National Council for the Blind and its constituent State and local bodies is supported by grants from central government. Rehabilitation courses that are available embrace daily living and communication skills, orientation and mobility, pre-vocational training and counselling, personal management, and crafts. Services such as these and the subsequent placement programmes for open and sheltered employment are available for blind members of the white, coloured, and black communities. In addition to

Rehabilitation and training

co-ordinating the work of 36 affiliated societies SANCB liaises with 37 associated organizations which provide direct services and ten State government departments. The work of the Council is supported through the payment of a block grant by the Department of Social Welfare and Pensions.

21

Employment and finance

Despite the remarkable and far-reaching progress that has been made in recent decades in the preparation and placement of blind people in an ever-widening range of occupations, trades, and professions, and notwithstanding the brilliant and well-publicized accomplishments of many blind men and women, the belief persists that blindness is synonymous with idleness and penury. If blindness strikes during working life, the man or woman concerned will probably imagine that it will be impossible to continue to do their job, raising the spectre of immediate and continuing unemployment and resultant poverty.

It is the accepted norm in modern society that all people will work, achieve a reasonable level of productivity, contribute to the economic strength of their communities, and through their own endeavours achieve a level of income sufficient to provide for the support of themselves and their families and enable them to enjoy the fruits of their labours in a variety of cultural leisure and recreational pursuits. Thus one of the first reactions of those who are afflicted by blindness may be fear that they will no longer be able to satisfy the norm expected of them and that sociologically as well as physically they will in future occupy a greatly reduced status in society and will be unable adequately to discharge their responsibilities to themselves and their families. Almost every type of employment initially appears to be wholly or largely dependent on the ability to see.

A tradition has grown up concerning the limited forms of work that can be performed by, or expected of, blind people. Some of the more traditional occupations do in fact continue to be performed to the present day and provide a useful level of income or serve a therapeutic purpose for a number of blind men and women. Even so, it is no longer the case that if a person becomes blind his future occupational life will consist of making baskets or brushes, hand knitting, weaving chair seats, or one of the other crafts based principally on manual dexterity that were the major occupations for blind people in days when work carrying regular remuneration was available only in the segregated setting of a special workshop for the blind. Later in this chapter it will be seen that prospects for productive, well-paid work are extremely bright if full advantage is taken of the resources currently available.

Finance

The twin spectres of idleness and poverty that haunt so many following the onset of blindness are closely related, and it must be admitted that the worry is not entirely ill-founded. Blindness can create considerable financial problems by causing unemployment or a down-grading of work leading to decreased income and by adding further financial burdens that impede effective rehabilitation.

For some journeys it may be necessary for the blind person to be accompanied by a guide. In most advanced countries, including those in North America, Australasia, South Africa, and Western Europe, provisions exist under which a blind traveller may be accompanied by a guide on main line trains upon payment of only one fare, although in the United Kingdom this privilege applies only after the purchase of a rail card which cost £10 annually when the scheme was introduced in 1981. However, blind people may travel to and from their schools or places of employment, or attend job interviews with a guide who travels free without the need to produce the rail card. In most advanced countries, travel concessions in respect of a blind person or his guide are available on most local and some long distance bus lines and underground or rapid transit systems. A number of internal airlines make similar arrangements for their blind passengers, but on most international routes the blind traveller and his companion must each pay full fare. Strenuous efforts are being made to persuade the International Air Transport Association to permit its members to offer concessions to blind travellers and their guides. Full fares must also be paid by escorts on most international shipping lines, although the members of the North Atlantic Conference and some others charge only half fare for the companion of a blind traveller.

In almost every area of daily life the blind person is at a financial disadvantage in direct comparison with his sighted counterpart and this can be a grave aggravation to his many other physical and psychological difficulties.

Blindness and visual handicap: the facts

Strenuous efforts have been made during recent years to persuade successive governments in the United Kingdom to adopt the practice already current in most of the advanced countries in Europe and elsewhere of paying to all registered blind adults a realistic blindness allowance designed to cover most of the unavoidable additional expenses incurred as a result of their blindness and regardless of income from other sources.

Through the inculcation of daily living techniques during rehabilitation, and the social service programmes provided by governments and private organizations, some ways have been found of reducing the level of additional cost imposed by blindness but, short of the introduction of a blindness allowance that would be received as a right by all blind adults, it seems likely that for the foreseeable future most people who become blind will find themselves forced to shoulder increased financial burdens.

Employment

Unless prevented by their age or very serious additional infirmity, most blind people of working age wish to take up, or resume, interesting and rewarding careers which utilize all their natural talents, and some may have undergone a course of rehabilitation or training for this purpose. However, during periods of acute economic depression, when large numbers of offices and factories are being closed, when the national level of unemployment is high, and substantial numbers of workers are being declared redundant, it is more difficult for blind and otherwise handicapped people to secure openings, and no cast-iron guarantee of employment can be offered to them. Nevertheless, specialized placements support is available, and in the United Kingdom all medium-sized and large employers are legally required to maintain on their payrolls a small percentage of disabled workers.

In most technically developed countries, the situation with respect to the employment of blind people has very much improved since the Second World War. Until that time, only a few blind people were engaged in professional careers such as lawyers, clergymen, musicians, and physiotherapists and the overwhelming majority of working blind people were employed on crafts such as basket and brush making, knitting,

164

boot and shoe repairing and other manual occupations in special work-shops for the blind. The extreme shortage of labour that was created throughout industry by the removal of millions of able young men and women for service in the Armed Forces created new opportunities for blind and other disabled workers and the success of the experiment created a firm foundation of confidence in the abilities of blind people which carried over into the post-war period and has since been further exploited. There came a growing realization that the skills of those who were blind need not be limited to repetitive manual tasks on the indus-trial shop floor but could extend to the executive, technical, adminis-trative, managerial, and clerical levels.

Governmental and voluntary action in a number of countries has led to the creation of assessment centres at which the skills and aspirations of young blind people, particularly those leaving school, could be evaluated and those concerned given full opportunity to become familiar with the broad range of possible career openings before committing themselves to any particular course. Such centres discharge a highly valuable function in enabling young blind people to set for themselves realistic career objectives.

In the United States, United Kingdom, Canada, Australia, New Zealand, and most other developed countries, central government bodies discharge the principal responsibility for funding or administering programmes for the placement of blind people in employment. Such activities are frequently conducted by national and local voluntary organizations who serve as the agents of government. Some of the functions thus discharged are conducting research into potential new areas of employment, the development and supply of technical aids which can be made available from government sources, the placement of blind men and women in industrial, commercial, administrative technical and professional occupations, and their placement in employ-ment or referral to appropriate further training courses.

The latest reviews of occupations being followed by blind or seriously visually handicapped persons indicate that during recent years there has been a steady trend away from blue-collar industrial employment into white-collar careers. Many new job opportunities have been opened up as a result of technological advances; for example the growth of the computer industry.

Blindness and visual handicap: the facts

The steadily increasing number of blind people who attend universities, other forms of higher and further education, and specialized training courses is resulting in larger numbers taking up professional and managerial careers, including university lecturers and all levels of the teaching profession. The practice of law continues to attract a number of blind candidates. More visually handicapped men and women are becoming qualified for, and taking up posts in many interesting areas of social work and whereas in past decades almost all were employed in programmes for the blind, most now become qualified as Technical Officers. The development of social services in recent years has meant that the majority of blind people now serve as generic social workers, carrying a mixed caseload and helping those suffering from a broad range of physical, mental, social, and financial deprivations. Others, including those who are located within hospitals, are serving successfully as medical or psychiatric social workers; thus the traditional place of blind people within the healing profession, so ably pioneered by very many blind masseurs and physiotherapists, is being consolidated. Many of today's blind physiotherapists are prepared through a curriculum offered at RNIB's new School of Physiotherapy, which admits trainees from a number of countries. They become fully qualified to handle with competence the range of complicated treatment equipment necessary in this age of advanced electrotherapy.

While there is a downward trend in the number of blind people who become clergymen or ministers of religion, a substantial number still practise the profession and new visually handicapped recruits to the priesthood continue to come forward. Doubtless because of the broadened range of professional opportunities now available to those without sight, fewer people than before enter the field of music, either as teachers or performers. However, the number who serve in a part-time capacity as church organists remains fairly constant and, of course, the value of music as a cultural and recreational pursuit for blind people, including those who are members of pop groups, cannot be over-stated.

The slight decline in the recruitment of the visually impaired to the clergy and music is counter balanced by the increasing numbers who gain high executive and administrative positions in general industrial and commercial life, salesmen, and those who satisfactorily own or manage small businesses of various types. Many enter and advance to ever-higher ranks within the public services; an increasing number are attracted to newspaper or radio journalism and other media of communication, and many work as clerks, braille shorthand and audio typists, and telephone switchboard operators.

The last of these occupations, which has served as a major source of employment for thousands of blind people, seemed a short while ago to be in danger of becoming a casualty of the technological age because certain switchboards which blind employees operated by touch were being replaced by boards which give visual signals and whose power source was too low to permit their adaptation for blind operators. However, as a result of a highly successful research and development programme funded by the National Research Development Corporation and undertaken at Imperial College, London, a prototype Conversion Kit using synthetic speech has been developed and fully tested by blind switchboard operators. A number of the conversion kits have already been installed.

Following the Second World War, the number of blind men and women working as operatives at many levels of industry, particularly as machine operators both in engineering and factories of other types, grew steadily. Such forms of open employment came to be regarded as the norm, and sheltered occupations, in special workshops for the blind, were often reserved for those who, for a variety of reasons, were considered to be unable to compete effectively with non-handicapped workers.

The ultimate objective of all rehabilitation programmes is to enable the visually handicapped to achieve the maximum level of integration, and to maintain a high level of open employment opportunities for those with limited sight. This has become more difficult due to the progressively higher level of automation within industry and the resultant decline in the total number of workers required to achieve a given level of production, together with the introduction of visual display techniques to control many of the processes for which in earlier times sight was not required. Together with these, the general problem of mass unemployment during a period of world and national recession has had an adverse impact on the employment of visually handicapped men and women in some occupations.

If jobs are to be found for all the visually handicapped people who are now available for placement, governmental and other resources will have to be fully utilized, and it is also extremely important that all those visually handicapped people who want to work should register their needs with the appropriate national, State, and local placement authority, or the voluntary body which serves as their agent. All employers should fully discharge their responsibilities by providing opportunities of employment to properly qualified blind men and women.

Despite the regrettable inroads that have occurred recently in the employment of blind people, a large number of blind workers continue to do a wide range of industrial tasks such as milling machine, capstan, lathe, drill and fly-press operators and as machine minders for many types of special-purpose engineering equipment. Blind operators have a good reputation in the woodworking, joinery, and other non-engineering trades, and current research in job development aims to evolve equipment and operating methods that will ensure a continuing place for blind workers in such areas of employment. Another example of open employment in the industrial world is the work of viewers and inspectors, and a number of special devices working to narrow tolerance, some providing audible output, have been designed for sightless operatives. Others work as warehousemen and store-keepers, and in a range of packing and labouring positions.

The steadily increasing number of blind people whose problems are additionally complicated by other physical or psychological defects, as well as those whose homes are in areas where little opportunity exists for vocational integration in open employment continues the need for work opportunities in special workshops for the blind and disabled. Such workshops have become more highly industrialized during recent years, with the installation of high-productivity equipment for the manufacture of a broadly increased range of products. The adverse economic situation in some countries has tended to increase the referral of blind people to special workshops.

It has not been our intention to list every form of work now open to people who suffer blindness or serious visual impairment. Sufficient examples have been quoted to indicate that, whatever the level of education or past experience, it is possible for most visually handicapped individuals to be satisfactorily resettled. Every effort should be made, through close collaboration between government departments, national and local voluntary bodies and organizations of blind people, to ensure that openings will be found which are consistent with the skills and aspirations of the affected individuals. It is confidently anticipated that, through further research and the evolution of more vocational equipment and devices, we shall move into a new era of job development, enabling blind people of working age to play their full and proper part in the economic life of the country.

At the end of Chapter 20, which dealt with rehabilitation and training, a brief review was given in the section entitled 'Government and voluntary services', of the programmes which exist in Australia, Canada, New Zealand, South Africa, the United Kingdom, and the United States, as a result of action that can be taken either directly by, or through collaboration between, governmental bodies and private organizations which serve the blind at the national, regional, or local level. The process of rehabilitation is an on-going one, embracing the provision of formal or 'on the job' training, and culminating in the placement of well adjusted blind men and women in suitable forms of employment for which they have been adequately prepared. In all the countries which have been mentioned, arrangements for the employment of blind people is undertaken by the same government departments and voluntary bodies as are involved in the provision of rehabilitation services and the operation of training schemes. For those wishing to be prepared for, or placed in, employment, full information can readily be obtained from the governmental and voluntary agencies to which reference has been made.

The blind person who has undergone the necessary rehabilitation and training, and has secured satisfying employment, will feel that life has begun anew, for once more he will experience the satisfaction of independent employment, and the knowledge that he has been restored to his proper role as a fully-participating and contributing member of his family and his community.

22

The elderly blind

Some 75 per cent of blind people in developed countries are beyond normal retirement age, so that in terms of numbers alone, blindness makes its greatest impact on the elderly. The full and active life which many younger blind people can enjoy may be beyond the physical capabilities of those whose visual handicap occurs in later life. The all-important senses of touch and hearing, so essential to the blind for the intake of information of all kinds, may have been blunted by the passage of years and so prove to be of only limited value.

Some people of advanced age master the intricacies of the braille code, but such cases are the exception rather than the rule. In those English-speaking countries where the Moon code is still practised a greater number of elderly blind people master that simpler system the reading of which is possible even when the sense of touch has been some-what impaired. Yet only a minority of those who become blind late in life achieve a level of tactile reading from which they can gain real satis-faction. For the rest, the intake of information and the pursuit of recreational 'reading' may well be limited to conversation, radio listening, Talking Books, Talking Newspapers, or other specially recorded material.

Similarly, loss of mobility can be rectified more easily in the young or middle-aged than in people of advanced years, few of whom will be able to take lengthy journeys on foot without assistance. As a result, many older blind people are dependent on others to take them out for walks if they are not to be confined indoors for long spells.

Elderly people should be encouraged to take an interest in what is going on around them. Yet this may not be fully recognized and, instead of helping them with the problems involved in keeping abreast of things, some well-intentioned helpers may genuinely, but wrongly, believe it unfair to expect them to undertake any activity involving strain, and an elderly person may be encouraged to sit quietly in a corner, be fed at appropriate intervals, and put to bed when the time comes, being occupied only with his thoughts or with memories of the past.

The elderly blind

At one time it was felt that the most appropriate way to overcome the difficulties faced by most visually handicapped old people was to accommodate them in special homes for the blind, some of which were founded and operated by charitable bodies. It is also commonly supposed that to expect younger family members to provide a home and extend all the supportive help that would inevitably be required to enable aging blind parents to live out their declining years in comparative comfort, might be an unjustifiable burden. Often the best answer for elderly folk is the provision of residence in a special home for the blind where the assistance of experienced and caring wardens and staff is readily available, where the companionship of other men and women with common interests and difficulties is at hand, and where layout, programmes, and equipment have been specially designed to minimize problems and enhance the enjoyment of life by blind people. But for some, the thought of abandoning their home is anathema, and many blind people fight resolutely for the opportunity to continue to live in the surroundings known and dear to them. Sometimes these wishes are overridden and a decision taken for residential care in the mistaken belief that blindness is a totally disabling condition and that those so affected must inevitably find themselves unable to take care of their own affairs, particularly if they are elderly.

Everything should be done to create a situation in which, despite blindness, an individual can achieve as closely as possible the pattern of life of his or her own choosing. Should he wish to remain in his own home, every possible assistance should be offered to help him to do so.

It cannot be denied that difficulties exist for elderly blind people, and not the least of these may be loneliness. Most of today's social workers and technical officers are well trained academically and many of them perform their caring tasks among elderly blind people with real understanding and helpfulness. On the other hand, the many problems of elderly blind people are not always fully appreciated by some generic social workers, and levels of service vary considerably.

Within the limits imposed by physical infirmity or emotional problems and the requirements of personal safety, efforts should be made by social workers who may be caring for older blind people and more especially by their relatives, friends, and neighbours to provide a level of support and assistance which will enable them to remain as active as

171

possible in mind and body, whether they are resident in a special home or continuing to live in their own surroundings. Many will wish to devote time to hobbies which they have previously pursued or to which they may be introduced; and in most instances methods exist through which the difficulties occasioned by blindness can be readily overcome. Some who have been keen gardeners will be able to continue with this interest despite the limitations of age and blindness, and in most countries national or local organizations for the blind are able to offer invaluable tips and simple gadgets which will ease the way for the visually handicapped gardener. Others may gain their greatest enjoyment from participating in the activities of men's clubs, women's institutes, church groups and the like, being prevented from doing so only by immobility resulting from age and blindness. With the expenditure of very little time and effort car-pools can be arranged to liberate elderly blind people from the confines of their everyday surroundings; and in the same way they can be helped to occasional attendance at musical events, theatres, local drama group productions, church services, and meetings of organizations.

The feeling of isolation which all too frequently accompanies old age is perhaps the most difficult for elderly people to overcome particularly when the additional factor of blindness is present. In such circumstances the telephone can act as a life-line, particularly at times of ill-health or other emergency. In most advanced countries governmental or voluntary programmes exist for the free installation of telephones in the homes of elderly blind people who are financially unable to make their own arrangements and it is hoped that this trend will continue. Being thus enabled to establish frequent voice contact with children, grand-children, and other loved ones, elderly blind people can escape at frequent intervals from the boredom of isolation. The tape recorder, too, can contribute immensely to that process, for it can serve as a means of correspondence between the elderly lonely blind person, and family members or friends even in other countries. The isolation of most elderly blind people can also be relieved by annual or semi-annual holidays; and while some will wish to share these with family members, or friends, at ordinary hotels or boarding houses, most national programmes for the blind maintain special holiday homes or hotels which may be purpose-built or adapted to present an easy lay-out for elderly people with visual impairment. At such establishments items of special equipment make life easier for the blind residents, while members of the staff are trained and experienced in the methods of assisting their blind guests to function happily in their temporary surroundings and extract the greatest enjoyment from their vacations.

By the methods described in this chapter and in a multitude of other ways, measures are available through which blind people of advanced years may be helped to savour the joy of living. With each passing generation the proportion of elderly people in our communities increases, as does the number of those who enter the later stages of life burdened by the handicap of blindness. It is the responsibility of all governments, national and local, as well as private bodies and individuals, to ensure that all possible steps are taken to alleviate the personal distress imposed on our senior citizens by this combination of difficulties.

23

Aids and devices

With the onset of blindness or serious visual impairment the affected person's ability to cope even with relatively simple facts of everyday life may be markedly reduced. With help from trained teachers and rehabilitation counsellors, some of the immediate effects can be ameliorated and the necessary adjustment made. However, the achievement of the total objective of active participation in normal actitivities will be accomplished only if a range of special aids and appliances is available. Devices which have been developed to overcome some of the problems most frequently encountered by blind people are discussed in this chapter.

Writing aids

The equipment for writing in braille ranges from a small pocket frame and stylus which can be used for jotting down notes, telephone numbers, addresses, and so on to the braille writing machine used for writing letters or any lengthy material. The braille frame or slate, whether pocket or desk size, consists of a series of cut-outs placed over a matched series of recesses. A piece of manila paper is placed between these two elements and braille symbols are formed when dots are pressed into the paper within the cut-out areas. Speedier writing can be achieved with the braille writing machine, as all the dots contained in any braille symbol are formed by one motion of the operator. The Stainsby braille writing machine developed in the United Kingdom has a flat base which can be placed on a desk or table surface, a guide fitted with six keys, and a space bar which can be used to form a complete line of braille before the guide is moved down to the next line. The braille produced in this fashion consists of dots pressed downwards into the paper, which has to be removed from the writing machine whenever the operator wishes to check what he has written.

The Perkins brailler was designed, developed, and is manufactured in the United States but is used throughout the world. It resembles a standard typewriter but with only the six keys and a spacer bar required to emboss the six dots of the standard braille cell. Paper is fed into the machine as for a normal typewriter. The Perkins machine differs from the Stainsby in two ways. First, it embosses only one side of the paper, whereas the Stainsby embosses on both sides with the dots on the second side falling between the lines or between the dots on the other side of the paper. Secondly, the Perkins punches the dots upwards so that the operator can read what he has written without having to remove the paper from the machine.

Machines of slightly different pattern, but performing the same function, are now being produced in many countries and full descriptions are readily available from the principal organizations serving the blind.

The Braille shorthand machine, manufactured in Britain, Germany, and elsewhere is a vital piece of equipment for the braille shorthand-typist or secretary, enabling him or her to emboss braille shorthand symbols at normal dictation speed on a spool of paper tape. The shorthand notes are later read by touch.

Many people who become blind are anxious to continue to write by longhand so that they can correspond with friends who are not blind. Most people retain legible handwriting for many years following the onset of blindness. The principal problem is keeping the lines straight, but this can be overcome in a variety of ways: the RNIB in the United Kingdom, the American Foundation for the blind in the USA, and similar organizations elsewhere, supply many types of handwriting guides. There are also special guides which enable blind people to sign documents and forms in the appropriate place.

Telling the time

Braille pocket watches and wrist watches are available. To tell the time, the blind user releases a spring catch which opens the lid or crystal cover, revealing the face of the watch marked with each hour. The hands of these watches are specially reinforced, and the blind user feels the time by running his fingers lightly over the two hands of the watch. A number of clocks have similarly been modified for touch reading; they have no glass front. Braille alarm clocks are in general use and the setting of the alarm can be easily accomplished by touch. A recent development has been the introduction of clocks and watches with synthetic speech output which announce the exact time to the user when a button is pressed.

Aids in the home

Many blind people utilize Braille timing devices that emit a clearly audible signal after the lapse of a selected length of time. This device is important in employment situations and to blind housewives for cooking. Other articles which can be of value in the kitchen or home include needle-threaders; label-making equipment for marking tinned goods and other items in the storeroom; an audible indicator which emits a bleep when tea or other liquid poured into a cup or container reaches the required level; jugs with embossed markings facilitating the accurate measurement of liquids; scales and balances for weighing ingredients; bread-cutting boxes, marked measures and rules which can be used for a variety of purposes; thermometers and barometers which can be read by touch; and a warning device which can be placed in the garden close to the washing line and emits a loud signal if it starts to rain. The controls of gas and electric cookers, washing machines, and other household equipment can be fitted with embossed marking.

Games

Playing cards and many other games and puzzles have been adapted for people who are blind, usually by adding braille dots. Playing pieces may be identified by their shape. Some examples of games which have been adapted in this way are chess, draughts, dominoes, lexicon, jig-saw puzzles, crossword puzzles, scrabble, ludo, and other similar games played with dice; additional games are introduced at regular intervals.

Special purpose aids and devices

Among the many pieces of equipment evolved for blind students and others, are physical and political maps produced in relief (usually in plastic material which withstands constant use), arithmetic and algebra frames, the Abacus compass and protractor. One of the more exciting developments of recent years is a calculating machine which, with the use of synthetic speech, can perform all the functions of a standard calculator. Numerous devices have been evolved to meet special situations. They include a sound beacon which emits an audible signal and can, for example, be attached to the handle of a lawn mower, enabling a blind gardener to return directly to it after emptying the grass container. Electronic light probes have many uses: they enable a blind person to locate a window or other light source within a room, to differentiate between dark and light clothing, to identify the location of a printed heading on writing paper, and to measure the intensity of light in a variety of situations.

There is a very broad spectrum of special aids for blind people in employment for example tools for carpentry; braille micrometers, depth gauges, and other precision engineering measurement devices (some with synthetic speech output); braille scales to facilitate control of margins and columns by blind typists, devices which enable blind music teachers to display staff notation and tonic solfa symbols to a class of sighted pupils; and the non-sighted equivalent of a spirit level with various uses in engineering and joinery.

Aids to mobility

The long cane, which can be obtained in rigid or folding form, is the means through which many blind men and women may be able to accomplish free and safe movement even on crowded streets, enabling them to detect danger points, safely negotiate steps up and down kerbs, uneven pavements, projecting building lines, and other hazards. The shorter guide and symbol canes serve the same purpose in part but their principal objective is to alert passers-by to the user's visual handicap so that they will be ready to lend a helping hand at street crossings or wherever the blind person is likely to meet with difficulties. If the blind user of a cane or stick also has a serious hearing defect, this is conventionally shown by marking the cane with a wide red band.

Unfortunately, some people with seriously failing sight regard the white stick with some abhorrence, as an indication of their total dependence on others and, in consequence, endeavour to manage without it for as long as they possibly can. I think they are misguided, and if they can once be persuaded to use this simple travel aid, they will find that in practice it has precisely the contrary effect, giving them a new and very rewarding level of independence.

Supplies of aids

All of the aids and appliances that have been described so far in this chapter and very many more can be obtained by blind people in the United Kingdom from the RNIB, local authority, Social Services Department, or local voluntary society for the blind. In the USA the principal supplier is the American Foundation for the Blind. The Canadian National Institute for the Blind, South African National Council for the Blind, and Australian National Council for the Blind, can provide details of similar equipment available in these countries.

The new technologies

One area of research in which a great deal of work has already been done is that of safe travel in the streets for blind people, and the science of ultrasonics has been used to develop environmental sensors which enable a blind user to receive, in tactile or audible form, more information about the immediate environment in which he is travelling than could be acquired through the use of even the longest cane. Some of the devices which are in use, or at the prototype stage, are mounted in canes of varying lengths; others are built into spectacle frames; some are carried on the chest; and others held in the hand. All use basically the same system: ultrasonic impulses are emitted and bounce back from obstacles which they strike. Those devices which have an audible output allow the blind user to form a sound picture of his immediate environment with the ability to detect and determine his distance from trees, lamp posts, solid and chain-link fences, building lines, other pedestrians, and moving traffic and to adjust his own movements accordingly. Those providing information in tactile form are held in the hand. The rate of output impulses enables the user accurately to estimate his distance from the object in his path.

At present most of these mobility devices are relatively expensive and another serious drawback is that, except in the case of those mounted in canes, it is not possible for the user to detect a step down. This means that for totally safe travel a blind person must use a long cane as well as wearing or carrying the ultrasonic guidance device. This is not very practical and considerable research effort is now being concentrated on overcoming the difficulty. If it is successful, the use of ultrasonic guidance devices by blind travellers may become common-place and the price of the appliance greatly reduced by the introduction of mass-production methods.

I referred earlier to the talking calculator, which uses synthetic speech. Sophisticated character-recognition equipment, perfected during recent years, has now been coupled with a synthetic speech output leading to the development and manufacture of machines which can read aloud. The first piece of equipment of this kind to come into pro-duction was invented in the United States and is known as the Kurzweil reading machine. This marked a breakthrough rivalling in potential importance the invention of the braille code. The machine can scan the printed pages of a book, line by line, recognize whole words or indi-vidual letters, figures, and punctuation and read the book aloud to a blind operator at whatever speed he may determine. The machine can recognize a number of different printing founts. In the United Kingdom the RNIB and St. Dunstan's (the British organization for blinded service men and women) acquired one of the earliest production models of this machine and during a period of evaluation many blind people have tested it and have been delighted to be able for the first time to read ordinary print directly. The quality of the spoken output, already quite acceptable, is being progressively improved and it is expected that the number of recognizable printing founts will be expanded.

The machines which are available to date can work effectively only with well-printed material so that poor carbon copies of typescript produce noticeably less good results. Similarly, the machine cannot yet decipher ordinary handwriting. In the years ahead it is likely that such drawbacks will be overcome and any blind person will in theory be able to read anything that has been produced in printed or written form. At present this equipment is extremely expensive and is thus out of reach of individual blind readers. The first step in the United Kingdom will probably follow that already taken in the United States; the installation of reading machines in a number of public libraries which serve relatively densely populated areas so that blind people can read, for example, selected study material or printed documentation required for vocational purposes. It is hoped that as demand grows, production will be improved and the cost reduced.

Whatever the future may hold with respect to the use of reading machines, it is clear that, for as far ahead as one can see, there will continue to be a need for the ever-increasing production of material in braille. In this regard the Kurzweil reading machine is a new boon to emerge from the technological age. The character-reading stage of the machine is now being marketed as the Kurzweil Data Entry Machine and is being used as an advanced technical process in the more rapid production of braille material. In brief, this machine reads from an ordinary printed book, converts it into digital form, and stores it on a magnetic tape. When this tape is fed through a computer, it can be used to motivate automatic transcribing machines which can either make a limited number of braille copies on manila paper or emboss the braille symbols on zinc plates which are used on printing presses for long-run production. Thus, the expensive and time-consuming stages of hand transcribing on zinc plates or key-punching material stored on tape are by-passed, and production of increased quantities of braille material is more rapid. This Data Entry Machine is already playing its part in a number of braille printing works.

The reading machine is unlikely to supplant all existing methods of touch-reading by blind people for some years to come, and in the meantime another product of modern technology will continue to be of considerable importance. It, too, works from the printed page, recognizing the shapes of letters and symbols and reproducing those shapes under the fingers of a blind reader by motivating clusters of vibrating pins. This machine is known as the Optacon (optical-to-tactile converter) and it is already proving of immense value to students and people in employment, enabling them to read printed material to which they could gain access in no other form. Short training courses in the operation of the equipment can be arranged in the United Kingdom by the RNIB and in other countries by national statewide organizations. In some instances individuals who require it for their jobs may secure one on permanent loan. Training is also being provided for pupils in educational programmes for the blind.

In one form or another, the computer is having its impact on our daily lives and it has become ever more necessary for means to be devised through which blind people can satisfactorily handle both the input and output stages, thus being able both to store and retrieve vital information which could be retained in no other manner. The specially devised machines serve in part as computer terminals, the input material being stored on magnetic tape cassettes and then being retrieved when required though the use of an indexing code enabling the machine to search the stored material, extract the required item, and present it in the form of a braille display for the blind user. At the point of presentation it replaces the conventional visual display unit used by sighted operators.

A considerable number of people become blind as a result of diabetic retinopathy, and it is necessary for them to monitor and control their blood sugar levels. For sighted diabetics this is a relatively simple technique, being based on the visual monitoring of colour change on a test strip dipped into a urine sample. Blind diabetics have to request others to conduct the urine test for them. Now, using modern microprocessing techniques, the blind person himself can monitor his condition. A small stick composed of a special chemical compound is placed in the urine container and an audible signal is emitted.

The future

Some decades into the future it may be possible for blind people to 'see' by means of synthetic or indirect vision. Several interesting research projects, particularly in the United Kingdom and the United States are already under way whereby through the medium of a miniaturized television camera, electronic impulses may be carried directly to the visual cortex of the brain, bypassing the eye and the optic nerve. Although such projects are now at only the initial and most tentative stage, sufficient evidence has already been acquired to justify the hope that it may be possible for blind people to gain, through direct stimulation of the brain, at least a hazy general concept of their surroundings and of items placed directly before the camera.

Neurological transplant technology may in the future reach a stage at which the transplantation of the whole eye will be possible, but it is unlikely that the authors or many of the readers of this volume will live to see that great day.

It is essential that theoretical and applied research projects should be maintained to look at the many areas of normal life which are affected by the loss of sight. Yet the cost of such research is high and economic factors are acting to decelerate the pace of progress in the United Kingdom. In certain countries, including Scandinavia, the Federal Republic of Germany, the United States, and some of the countries of Eastern Europe, considerable government funds are now being channelled into medical and technical research relating to blindness, whereas in Britain the majority of such activities must be funded by charitable bodies or individual benevolence, even if the research is done in universities or hospital departments. Britain has always held a greatly respected position as one of the world's leaders in this area of humanitarian activity and it would be sad indeed if she were forced to relinquish her place. We believe that government funds should be made more freely available.

Low vision aids

When someone suffers serious visual loss from any cause the sight that remains can very often be improved by what are known as Low Vision Aids (LVA). These are usually magnifying devices of various kinds and their effect can often be enhanced by adjusting the lighting conditions or improving the contrast; for example using colour rather than black and white.

There are no hard-and-fast rules about what device suits any one patient best; often variety is used for different functions. Throughout the United Kingdom there is an increasing number of LVA clinics, usually found in district or ophthalmic hospitals (but some privately run) in which highly trained opticians, partly by calculation and partly by experience, select and prescribe the aids that best improve the vision for the purpose required by the patient.

In order to improve the distance vision some sort of telescopic device is needed. This may be binocular (up to $\times$ 5) or monocular (up to $\times$ 9) and either hand-held or fixed to a spectacle frame. The magnification is adjustable. They are particularly useful for viewing a small area such as a television screen, fishing float, or bus number but no use for general mobility as the field of vision is very restricted.

Aids for near vision are in general more useful. The main points to be decided are whether it is necessary for both hands to be free, as for sewing, and if it is to be used for reading, whether this is to be for pleasure or for information. The most useful and the cheapest device is the humble magnifying glass, but this leaves only one hand free. Although the magnification can be as high as × 10 or more there is the great snag that the field of view is restricted to a few words and the patient easily tires of the exercise. It is therefore often better to sacrifice magnification and to have a wider field. However, when it comes to reading for information: reading a letter, looking up a telephone number, or attending to other details where one does not want to be dependent on others, the hand magnifying glass is a great boon.

Large-print books designed for the partially sighted are available in most libraries but the avid reader may find the selection of titles available rather restricted.

Spectacle magnifiers, which allow both hands to be free, are either made as binocular or monocular aids. The latter are in general more useful. The simple expedient of giving a reading addition of 5 or 6 dioptres instead of the usual 3 dioptres for the elderly often greatly enhances the use of ordinary reading glasses and if only the better eye is used and the weaker blacked out, the shorter reading distance is not too great a strain for most. Other types of spectacle magnifiers are made on the telescopic principle and enable the patient to hold the book or close work at a more normal distance. They give a magnification of × 9 (monocular) or × 5 (binocular). The former is in general more useful. These little telescopes have standard threads so that if the vision continues to deteriorate higher powers can be obtained simply by screwing them in, without the necessity of buying new frames.

The highest magnification, which sometimes allows those on the full blind register to read for information, is obtained by closed circuit television (CCTV). This will give a magnification of × 50. The equipment is a little difficult to manage, and very expensive at present.

Good illumination is essential for LVAs. The light source should be behind the patient, over the left shoulder in right-handed people. This ensures that the light is reflected *away* from the patient's eyes. The optimum intensity must be found by trial and error. In most cases the brighter the light the better and a metal shade delivers most light. However, there are exceptions; where, for example, the impaired vision is caused by a central cataract a very bright light will constrict the pupil and thus actually reduce the vision.

24

Trail-blazers

In the modern world those who are blind can face life with the confidence that springs from personal and public recognition of their level of competence — but this did not happen purely by chance. From time to time throughout history there have emerged sightless individuals who planted the seeds from which today's harvest of practical support and understanding have sprung. So, as we press on with our task of further extending the horizons of the blind it is appropriate that we should pause to offer our gratitude to a few of the outstanding blind pioneers of earlier days.

Homer

The name of Homer will live forever as perhaps the world's greatest classical writer of epic verse. Such would have been the case because of his dazzling insight and the incomparable merit of his masterpieces the *Odyssey* and the *Iliad*; but for those who are particularly interested in the subject of blindness his work must assume an even higher level of significance and he will forever be revered as one of the towering figures of exemplary attainment.

It is disappointing that the facts of his early life, the age at which blindness occurred, and the cause of his visual defect — and even the precise date of his birth — are uncertain. It is believed that he was born in Smyrna about 850 BC into a family whose financial circumstances enabled him to achieve a high level of education. Certainly his subsequent life pattern indicates a passionate interest in literature and the construction of classical verse: also of geography and the effect of cultural patterns on community behaviour.

He travelled extensively through the lands of the Greek Empire bordering the Mediterranean and had undoubted influence on the development of Classical schools of thought and literature in the lands that were touched by his travels and his personality. It is widely believed

185

that he became blind while travelling through Ithica and it is known that he established a School of Poetry in Chios. His fame spread before him through the countries and the islands of the area and when he was shipwrecked on the Island of Samos, the thinkers and distinguished men of the period welcomed him to their homes as an honoured guest. Tradition has it that his life and work ended at Ios where he was buried. The perceptivity and strength of Homer's work ensures his permanent place as the great master of historic verse and it is unlikely that the Odyssey will ever be surpassed as the creative product of the mind of a blind genius.

Didymus of Alexandria

Didymus of Alexandria, who lived in the 4th century AD, provides perhaps the first instance of a full and well-rounded education being gained by a blind child and utilized to the full in an immensely valuable lifetime of service as a pre-eminent thinker of his day. Born in 308 and blind before reaching the age of five, he displayed an indomitable spirit and insatiable thirst for knowledge, coupled with an agility of mind which enabled him to overcome the most daunting difficulties. He early learnt the shapes of the letters of the alphabet and arranged for wooden letters to be carved which he used to good effect in forming words, phrases, and sentences. While this system served as the basis of his early self-instruction, it was only a means to an end.

Soon he had gathered around him a group of readers who brought to his receptive mind the enlightenment he was seeking from the scrolls and writings of that and earlier ages. He quickly gained skills in literary endeavour and on theological subjects, developing to the point at which he ultimately became a Professor of the University of Alexandria, then one of the world's most distinguished centres of learning. Like so many blind people, before and since, he was a highly talented musician, while he also won renown in the fields of mathematics, philosophy, and astronomy.

A student of rhetoric, his dissertations were said to have been delivered with tremendous force and clarity and among the people whose lives he profoundly influenced may be numbered St. Anthony, who became such a great figure in the early growth of the Christian Church,

186

and St. Jerome, who later was to be revered as one of the Four Doctors of Early Christendom. Didymus died in the year 395 but the example he set, and the influence he wielded, are with us still.

St. Hervé

The story of St. Hervé, who was born in Brittany probably towards the end of the 5th century, provides an early but somewhat brief record of an outstanding blind person emerging in Western Europe. The son of a bard who was held in high esteem, St. Hervé was either born blind or lost his sight in early childhood. He quickly developed a great affinity for music to which he was doubtless introduced by his father and to the Christian faith to which his mother had earlier been converted. His unique ability with song and instrument, together with his piety in spreading the Christian message, gained him considerable renown in Northern France during his lifetime and these two facets of his character were to win him a place in the history of the world.

He founded in Brittany a small monastery where he devoted his musical talents to the furthering of his Christian beliefs and in due time that monastery was to become a permanent shrine held in the deepest reverence by all blind musicians. Even today the Feast of St. Hervé is celebrated each June with a gathering of blind musicians from all over France and other countries in a service of thanksgiving and rededication. The pilgrims bring their musical instruments with them, calling upon St. Hervé to bestow his blessing and to add sweetness to the music they produce.

Many of the blind people who participate in these ceremonies are led by guide dogs and in this also they are marking the footsteps of St. Hervé himself for tradition has it that in his travels throughout Brittany and Northern France he, too, was led by a dog. St. Hervé died in 565 but his memory lives on being enshrined in his role as the patron saint of all blind musicians.

Prince Hitoyasu of Japan

Prince Hitoyasu of Japan was born in the year 843 to a life of luxury and power. His father, the Emperor of Japan, arranged his complete education and training and public administration in order that he could play his full role as a capable and understanding leader of the nation. Blindness struck in Prince Hitoyasu's twenty-eighth year by which time he was serving as Governor of two Provinces of the country. Much can be learned of the character of the man that he did not permit this personal tragedy to overwhelm him, nor did he simply retire to the life of comfort and ease that his financial circumstances would have permitted.

During his early education he had gained a deep interest in poetry and music so that after the onset of blindness he was convinced that he could serve an invaluable function both by furthering these arts and by encouraging and assisting all blind people to find appropriate outlets for their talents. Accordingly he gathered around him in his court at Kyoto a group of blind people drawn from all parts of the country, in order that he could familiarize himself with their circumstances, their difficulties, and their aspirations. He found that many, like himself, had an inherent talent for music and under his patronage the Court at Kyoto became a centre of music instruction and performance for blind people while he himself gained the warmest approbation for his own musical and poetry recitals. He learnt, too, that the delicate touch sense of blind people could be utilized to the advantage of the people of the country through the practice of massage.

As a result of his representations on these points, it was decreed by his father, the Emperor, that the practice of music and massage as professional occupations should be reserved for blind people, thus bringing to many of his contemporaries a new level of financial security. This was probably the first occasion in history when certain appropriate occupations were specially scheduled or reserved for practice by those with physical infirmities, a practice which continues until today. Similarly, the special place of blind people in the fields of music and massage has continued to be observed in Japan where special music academies and training centres in massage, acupuncture and moxi-cautery still exist exclusively for the benefit of those without sight.

Abdul ala al Maarri

Abdul ala al Maarri was born in Aleppo in the year 973. He lost his sight at the age of four, a victim of smallpox which was then a scourge to the health of the whole of the Middle East. Little is known of his early life but it may be presumed that he came from a wealthy family which was able to arrange for him to work with tutors who provided instruction by word of mouth. Abdul had an aesthetic nature, a quick and enquiring mind, and a desire to absorb and retain all the knowledge reaching him through his ears. There seems little reason to doubt the reputation he gained for prodigious feats of memory, it being said of him that his thirst for more and more knowledge remained unquenched despite his fabulous accomplishment in memorizing the total contents of all the books in the libraries at Haleb, Antioch, and Tripoli.

Very early his principal interest became centred in poetry and his writings in verse were of such quality that when he visited the fabulous city of Baghdad in the year 1008 he found himself welcomed as the honoured guest of all the literary figures of the age. His work ushered in a new era in the poetry of the region, for the first time concentrating principally on the quality of life and the need for all to make quest for spiritual objectives. It is generally accepted that his work marked the zenith of the Age of Poetry in the Persian Empire and the philosophies which he so ably expounded in his writings continue to be respected to this day.

Johann Ziska

History is replete with stories of brave men who have lost their sight in battle but it is seldom indeed that a person so sorely wounded has been able to soldier on and to win a new and envied reputation as a blind Leader and General.

One such case occurred in the Middle Ages in Bohemia where Johann Ziska, born late in the fourteenth century, was a greatly feared and able General. He lost one eye in battle against the Poles and the other in the field at Prague. Yet, despite blindness, he continued to lead his troops and was armed with a poleaxe which it is said he used to great advantage, both in attack and as a means of transmitting signals to his troops. His skill in strategy and manoeuvre became legendary, and it was said that he was more greatly dreaded by his enemies after he became blind than before.

Blindness and visual handicap: the facts

He was known to be a learned man and unmatched in his age for detailed knowledge of the geographical features and terrain of the countries of Central Europe. The skill and courage that he displayed as a fighter, his complete adjustment to the totally changed circumstances imposed by blindness particularly in his chosen profession, his academic attainments combined with his political qualities as a reforming leader of Bohemia gave him a permanent place in the histories of warfare, of European political development and the accomplishments of the blind.

John Milton

John Milton (1608–74), one of the brightest blossoms in the bouquet of English and world poetry, is rightly revered for his glittering accomplishments as a writer of classical verse following the onset of blindness. However, his total loss of sight did not occur until he had achieved middle age, although there is strong evidence to indicate that he suffered from severely impaired vision for most of his life.

It is likely that his love of verse was nurtured by his father, a writer of madrigals, and that the eloquence of his descriptive poetic style matured during a lengthy Classical education at St. Paul's School, London and Cambridge University.

He spent seven years at Cambridge University, possibly because of difficulties imposed on his studies by the progressive diminution of his sight but they were years which won for him a reputation throughout Europe as a distinguished scholar, whose classical and artistic attainments provoked universal interest and praise. This was clearly evident from the warmth of the welcome extended to him when he made the Grand Tour of Europe after leaving the university, by which time he had already commenced work on his sonnets. The great Galileo was already blind when Milton met him on his journeyings and it is interesting to speculate whether one of his reasons for seeking the meeting may have been the desire to exchange views about the problems of living with impaired vision.

After returning to England, Milton devoted much of his time to political endeavour, including the publication of many pamphlets principally in support of the Republican cause. He was an outspoken admirer of Oliver Cromwell and was the centre of considerable political controversy as a result of his writings. Later Cromwell was to reward him for his unflagging work as a pamphleteering campaigner, by appointing him Secretary of State for Foreign Tongues in the government he formed after the removal of Charles I from the throne.

It was after the total loss of sight occurred at the age of 44 that Milton fully developed the creative and inspirational talent which has caused his work to be universally acclaimed. *Paradise Lost*, *Paradise Regained*, and *Samson Agonistes* all flowed from the brilliant mind of a man already bereft of sight. *Paradise Lost*, published in 1677, was written in a cottage at Chalfont St Giles in the Buckinghamshire countryside and the small house is still maintained in the care of a Trust as a museum and shrine to this great blind Master of the past.

Nicholas Saundersson

Nicholas Saundersson was born in Yorkshire, England, in 1682 and became blind at the age of one following an attack of smallpox. To that time there had been few examples in England of the acquisition of significant levels of education by blind children but, clearly, Saundersson's parents had an enlightened attitude and resolved that their son should not grow up in ignorance. Nicholas's father laboured lovingly to teach him arithmetic and to introduce him to the glories of literature, even arranging for his admission as a blind child to the small local school. The boy's progress seemed to be so promising that before long arrangements were concluded for him to attend a private educational Academy in nearby Sheffield.

Having earlier familiarized himself with the shapes of letters and numbers, he made rapid progress displaying an astounding ability for rapid mental calculation. He devised for his personal use a number of ingenious devices which permitted him to master complicated arithmetical, algebraic, and geometrical problems, such equipment being the fore-runners of the arithmetic frames and mathematics devices still in widespread use by the blind today and only recently supplemented by electronic calculating machines. The immense ability which he displayed as a result of his studies in Sheffield so impressed the Academicians of the day that he was permitted to attend Cambridge University, not as a full student but with uninhibited access to the library, a concession which he utilized to the fullest advantage.

Blindness and visual handicap: the facts

This was the period when the whole world of learning was struggling to understand and evaluate the revolutionary new theories being advanced by Sir Isaac Newton and despite his blindness, coupled with the totally abstract nature of the Newtonian principles, including their concentration on light and colour, Saundersson soon emerged as one of the very few who could both understand and expound on the theories with total clarity. Naturally this was welcomed excitedly by Newton himself, who became Saundersson's patron, taking a personal interest in his career and helping in his academic advancement. Soon Saundersson had become a tutor at Cambridge University, specializing in teaching Newtonian principles and as a result of the influence of Sir Isaac's persuasive pressure on Queen Anne, a Degree was conferred on Saundersson enabling him before reaching the age of 30 to be appointed Lucasian Professor at Cambridge. Honours continued to be heaped on him through the rest of his regrettably short life, including his admission as a Fellow of the Royal Society in 1719 and the conferment of the Degree of Doctor of Laws by King George II.

Most of Saundersson's days were spend in the sedentary life of an Academician and in the often lonely dissemination of knowledge, yet he is known to have been a man of wit as well as intellect, a forceful and effective lecturer and without doubt one of the greatest blind scholars of all time. He died in 1739 of scurvy at the age of 57.

John Metcalfe

Born in a village near Knaresborough in Yorkshire, England, in the year 1717, John Metcalfe was to become one of those blind people whose lives are full of energetic achievement in the world outside the halls of learning and in the more physical and competitive fields of commerce, engineering, and adventure. Becoming blind in his sixth year, Metcalfe was, nevertheless, known to have enjoyed rude physical health becoming an expert horseman and strong swimmer.

From an early age he tramped the roads, hills, and dales of the surrounding countryside, travelling alone and aided only by a stout staff. His skill in personal mobility would have been envied by many blind people of today whose travel horizons remain circumscribed, for

192

Metcalfe became a familiar figure throughout the North of England. Blind Jack of Knaresborough, as he was familiarly known, built up a broad range of business interests and commercial ventures all over the North and Midlands of England, maintaining personal supervision of his business empire by almost constant journeying. But his life was not all energy and muscle. Music, too, was one of his abiding interests and he was an accomplished player of wind instruments. This interest, combined with his natural sense of adventure to cause him to join the English troops as they met in battle the Scots and as a musician he served in the field during more than one historic battle.

During his travels, on foot and by horseback, Metcalfe suffered many discomforts largely due to the deplorable condition of most roads at that time and determined to improve the situation. In the years that followed he negotiated numerous contracts for road construction and is credited with responsibility for the introduction of the practice of using crushed stone to provide a durable surface to withstand wear and weather. In the process of linking towns with new roads, Metcalfe had to overcome many problems of terrain and in the process became a skilled bridge-builder. In the life of this remarkable and self-taught man is to be found an inspirational story of determination, personal adjustment, ingenuity, and the full enjoyment of life.

Francois Huber

In Switzerland in 1750 was born Francois Huber who was a victim of cataracts and suffered from defective sight during his infancy and boyhood and became totally blind before his sixteenth birthday. Yet his fame will live on as one of the memorable blind people of the world, having achieved outstanding feats of discovery and scientific deduction in the unlikely field of bee keeping.

The son of a soldier who was a friend of Voltaire, Francois attended lectures at the University of Geneva but being the victim of consumption he was forced to discontinue these studies in order to satisfy his doctor's urgent recommendations that he should live in the countryside. Having married his childhood sweetheart Maria, the new family home was established in the country and so began the observation and scientific study of the life cycle, habits, structure and community organization of the hives, and honey-making activities of bees. It was almost entirely through the detailed observations and deductions of Huber, ably assisted by Maria, that a total fund of knowledge has been built up to the great advantage of all subsequent generations of apiarists.

As they worked together, matters that had previously been shrouded in mystery became clear, with scientific proof evolving from theoretical deduction on such matters as the reasons for swarming, the life cycle of the queen bee, her impregnation while in flight away from the hive, the ventilation of sealed hives through the wing action of its residents and the full process of honey-making and storage.

Huber's meticulous scientific observations and accurate deductions paved the way to the publication of his findings in 1792 and none of his judgments have proved to be misplaced in nearly two centuries of further study that has occurred since that revealing document was given to the world. Like so many other blind men and women, known and unknown, Huber found a special relaxation in music. He displayed a gentle urbanity and until his death in 1831 shared a loving relationship with Maria, his ever present partner at work and in the home.

Maria von Paradis

The opulence, splendour and gaiety of the eighteenth-century royal courts of Europe provided the background to the fascinating life of the charming Maria von Paradis, who was born in Vienna in 1759, the daughter of a Counsellor at the Court of Empress Maria Theresa. A happy outgoing child, Maria was the apple of her parents' eyes and a pampered plaything in Court and society circles. Then at the age of three she was stricken with a seizure which left her totally blind. The ministrations of the leading oculists and other medical specialists of Europe proved unavailing as did later a prolonged course in mesmerism at the controversial clinic Mesmer had established.

Maria was a bright and energetic child and under the tutelage of teachers specially obtained for her with the help of the Empress, she soon began to blossom, achieving a creditable level of proficiency in languages, history, and geography, all required subjects for one who moved in the high society circles of that day. She learnt to move confidently from place to place, was a graceful dancer and by the age of

194

nine was displaying the deep interest in and unusual talent for music that was later to win her popular acclaim throughout the continent. When she sang before Empress Maria Theresa, during a concert at St. Augustine's Church when she was twelve years old, the Queen was so favourably impressed that she became her patron and arranged for Maria to receive training in voice and piano at the hands of the leading musicologists of the Court.

Within a few years the name of Maria von Paradis became a household word throughout Europe, for not only had she proved herself to be a brilliantly accomplished singer and pianist but also a gifted conversationalist and dancer, a happy and beautiful young girl with a friendly outgoing disposition, who moved easily in all circles of society where she was welcomed as a brilliant star on the social and musical scene. Before long she set off on her travels through Europe, where she won the hearts of all just as she had done in her homeland.

She had been endowed with virtually all of life's blessings, save the gift of sight, and it was her constant concern that, despite the undoubted progress that had been made towards providing the sightless with the means of maintaining life, most of them still had no means of securing education. At each capital city, where her concerts were received enthusiastically, she made enquiries about the condition of blind people, meeting many of them to discuss their circumstances and difficulties and encouraging the influential to take forthright action to improve the situation.

On a tour of France in 1784, she achieved glittering success on the concert stage and played the piano and sang for Marie Antoinette in the Palace at Versailles. There she met Valentin Hauy, who had for a number of years been planning to introduce educational opportunities for blind children, and to him Maria von Paradis described her own determined attitudes concerning the mass education of the blind. Later that year Hauy was to open the world's first school for blind children and so to launch the modern era of education for the sightless. That he did so may be ascribed in a certain measure to the example set by Maria von Paradis and to the intensity and persuasiveness of the arguments she advanced, for later Hauy wrote that at the time of their meeting he was besieged by doubts but that his conversations with Maria had restored his confidence to proceed.

During her meeting with Hauy, Maria von Paradis drew to his attention the achievements of a young blind man in Mannerheim named Weissemburg with whom she had, with difficulty, engaged in some correspondence by pin-prick writing. He had first approached her in similar fashion to tell of the inspiration she had brought to his own studies under Christian Niesen, as a result of which, with the assistance of the peg-board and other devices evolved by Saundersson in England and using embossed maps of his own devising, he had gained high proficiency in a very broad range of classical, mathematical, and scientific subjects as well as music and the arts. Here was yet more evidence to Hauy of the unlimited world of learning that could be opened to those without sight. The incident, too, serves as an early example of the influence that blind people can bring to bear, by co-operation between each other and with those who can see, towards the planning and delivery of essential programmes for the education and social betterment of the blind.

During her tour of Europe Maria von Paradis visited England where she was received at Windsor Castle by the Prince of Wales, later to become King George II, for whom she sang and with whom she engaged in duets, he performing on cello and she on piano. At the end of her tour she returned to Vienna and throughout the rest of her life gained the plaudits of her audiences by the brilliance of her musical presentation, while continuing to keep alert to the special needs of the blind and to influence others towards the introduction of well planned services. But her music was her greatest gift to the age in which she lived and it gained the admiration of all her audiences, including the composer Mozart who dedicated a concerto to her. Maria was a composer in her own right having written a number of operas which were performed in Vienna and elsewhere but, unhappily, never published. She died in 1824 at the age of 64.

Louis Braille

Louis Braille, the inventor of the unique, all-embracing, yet comparatively simple system of reading and writing, the greatest single factor in the world-wide emancipation of blind people, was born in the small town of Coupvrey some 23 miles from Paris on 4 January in the year

1809. The son of a saddler and harness maker, his birthplace was a typically small country house where he, his three brothers and sisters, and parents resided and where his father maintained his workshop.

As a very small boy Louis enjoyed watching his father working with leather and it was shortly before his fourth birthday that the accident occurred that was to cost Louis his eyesight. He was trying his own hand at piercing a hole in a strip of leather with an awl when the tool slipped and pierced an eye. The sight of that eye could not be restored and before long an infection had settled in the other one plunging Louis into the world of darkness in which he was to remain throughout his life.

Although he was a shy, somewhat reserved lad he soon began to learn to fend for himself, to wander the fields and lanes of the area and to venture into the busy market place in the little town to which he later brought such eminence. His youthful intelligence and persistence were noted by the local schoolmaster and soon he was admitted to a class there where, unable to read or write, he learnt by rote and was soon seen to have a thirst for knowledge which could not easily be assuaged.

It was probably the death of Louis's father in 1819 that led to the decision to send him to the School for the Blind in Paris as a means of reducing financial strain on the family now that the harness-making business was no more. When he passed through its portals later that year a new vista of hope and opportunity opened up before the boy from Coupvrey and he grasped eagerly at the chance that fate had afforded. Within a year he had won the special attention of his teachers as a boy of great promise and innate ability and he revelled quietly in the joy that he extracted from music and the broadened academic curriculum he could now follow.

As the years passed he became particularly skilled, as a cellist and organist, being appointed in his teens to be Organist Intern at the Church of St. Nicholas in the Fields and the more important church of St. Vincent de Paul. It was during this period, however, that he developed the symptoms of lung infection which over the succeeding years were so frequently to interrupt his studies and his work in order that he could return to Coupvrey to be nursed back to health by his mother.

When the time came for Louis to leave the Paris school, he was requested to stay on as an assistant teacher and in 1828, at the age of 19, he became a full Professor of the establishment. It was a very unusual thing for a blind person to serve as a teacher at the school, but it soon became apparent that Louis's own personal knowledge of the problems posed by lack of sight, and his ingenuity in overcoming them, added greatly to his value as an instructor during the classes he conducted in history, geometry, and algebra.

Taking his teaching duties seriously Louis recognized that, despite his best efforts, the educational attainments of his pupils would always remain proscribed until the blind had full and unlimited access to books and the ability to refer to their own notes. He was, therefore, greatly intrigued when he became aware of a system of embossed dots and lines on paper which had been evolved some years earlier by a Charles Barbier, an Army officer, as a silent means of passing messages between military units at night. Over the years Barbier had evolved a number of modifications to his original system but it had not been recognized as being of potential value to the blind. In fact, when Barbier's code finally reached the school at which Louis was employed, the headmaster decided that it was of little consequence and set it aside. However, when it came to Louis's attention he recognized its potential. The code which Barbier had then devised was rapidly adjudged by Louis Braille to be deficient in a number of respects. Firstly, it consisted basically of a grouping of twelve dots, the size of each group being such that it could not be covered by a single finger-tip. Furthermore, the rules for deciphering the groupings were far too numerous and complicated.

Having obtained Barbier's permission to modify the system in any manner that might make it suitable for use by the blind, Louis Braille set to work. His first step was to eliminate all the embossed lines and to reduce the groupings of dots to a maximum number of six set down in two parallel lines of three. Thus emerged the braille 'cell' which was, and still remains, the basis for the braille code. A special slate was devised which simplified the process of embossing dots on the paper using a stylus whose shape was fatefully similar to that of the awl which had caused Louis Braille's blindness. It remained for the 63 combinations of dots achievable in a six-dot cell, each to be assigned a value as a letter, punctuation mark, numeral, letter grouping or word and the Code developed by Braille proved to be a masterpiece of orderly simplicity.

This was the achievement for which blind people had been waiting since the beginning of time. The system was now at hand by which any book could be printed in a form that could be read by those without sight. Here was a method which enabled blind people to make their own notes, to correspond with each other even at great distances, to make their own calculations, to keep their own accounts — in short, to remove the obstacles that had barred their way to education and progress.

By 1834 the braille code had been completed, including its utilization for writing musical notation, but the authorities of the Paris school were slow to recognize the immense significance of what had been accomplished by their young blind teacher and Braille was forbidden to introduce the system into the classroom, although he was permitted to teach it to blind pupils in his own time. This he did and his efforts were greeted with gleeful enthusiasm by those pupils of the Paris School who were fortunate enough to be in residence at the genesis of this historic breakthrough. Following the publication, by Braille, of a pamphlet in 1839 in which the braille system was described in full detail, with generous credit being given to Charles Barbier for his early work in a pioneering role, general interest increased but the sighted administrators of Braille's school continued to be lukewarm and it was not until 1850 that it was officially introduced as a teaching medium.

Louis Braille did not live to see the fruits of his labours sweeping across the world to liberate blind people from the bonds of ignorance that had enslaved them in past generations. His lung condition worsened, no doubt accelerated by the long days and nights he had spent in perfecting his sytem of reading and writing, and he was forced to return to Coupvrey in an effort to arrest the illness. He died there on 16 January 1852 at the age of 43, and was buried in the town churchyard.

By 1887 he had become a great figure in the history of the world and an impressive monument to his memory was erected in the market square which was renamed Place Braille. In 1952, on the hundredth anniversary of his death, the citizens of France and the blind people of the world paid their homage to the great emancipator. His remains were removed from the simple grave at Coupvrey to rest for ever at the Pantheon in Paris alongside the other great men and women of the land.

Blindness and visual handicap: the facts

Behind his bier, as the cortege wound solemnly through the streets of Paris, marched a huge company of blind people who had travelled from the ends of the earth to give public testimony to their indebtedness to their hero. He will live for ever in the hearts and in the lives of all who are blind. Yet he still remains a part of Coupvrey for, when his body was exhumed for reinterment in the Pantheon, the hands which had fashioned and had been the first to read the miraculous braille code were left undisturbed, so they will remain for all time close to the revered birthplace now maintained by the blind people of the world as a permanent memorial to their liberator.

Thomas Rhodes Armitage

In the decades that immediately followed the development of Braille's reading system for the blind, a number of alternative codes were devised with some of them securing considerable support. This created a potentially explosive situation since there was great danger that, short of learning all the codes, a blind person's reading would be restricted to the literature which happened to be produced in the code with which he was familiar. Thus developed what has come to be known as the 'battle of the dots' during which the proponents of rival codes sniped at each other and fought long and hard to gain the broadest acceptance of the particular code which they favoured.

One of the most ardent and successful supporters of the Braille Code was Dr Thomas Rhodes Armitage who was born in the County of Sussex in Southern England in 1824. A handsome, energetic man who was deeply interested in helping mankind Armitage was drawn to medicine as a career and after completing his studies at King's College in London he was admitted as a Member of the Royal College of Physicians. Despite having had defective vision from his youth, he went on to develop a successful London practice and his personal experience of visual defect may have caused him to take a particularly deep interest in one of his patients whose declining sight ultimately led to blindness. Later this proved to be Dr Armitage's own fate for his own vision became steadily more impaired until in 1860 he was forced to give up the practice of medicine and to start a new life as a blind person.

In his youth he had travelled and studied extensively in Europe and had become aware of the burgeoning movement throughout the Continent for the education of blind people. In addition, the enquiries he had made on behalf of his blind patient had led to his familiarizing himself with the braille code and some of the alternative systems that were being advanced. Thus when his own blindness forced a change of career, he resolved to dedicate the rest of his life to improving the circumstances of the sightless in Britain and abroad. He swung rapidly into action, visiting the blind people in their homes, persuading some of his influential friends to take relief action. He travelled to the Continent to study the work of the School for Young Blind in Paris and similar establishments in other countries. What he saw left him with certain unshakeable convictions, one of which was that the braille code was unsurpassed as a reading and writing medium for blind people and he, thereafter, became one of its most powerful advocates.

In 1868 he founded the British and Foreign Blind Association which in due time was to develop into today's Royal National Institute for the Blind, one of the world's most powerful, influential, and successful national organizations for the provision and progressive improvement of programmes for the education, rehabilitation, training, employment, cultural, and leisure pursuits for blind people of all ages. The production of embossed literature in the braille code for the benefit of visually handicapped people in Britain and elsewhere was a primary object of the new organization and Armitage launched far-reaching international action to ensure that the braille system should gain primacy. That such ultimately proved to be the case was due in large measure to the persuasive vehemence with which Armitage presented his case and as the years passed the predecessor organizations of RNIB were able to publish an ever-growing quantity of braille material to meet the mounting demand from English-speaking and other countries of the world.

But the acceptance and publication of braille was far from being Armitage's sole interest as he approached his new tasks on behalf of blind people. He displayed an unshakeable confidence in the ability of the sightless to play an important part in the organization of their own affairs and to participate in the development of policies which would have a bearing on their lives. He insisted that all of the members of the founding Committee of the British and Foreign Blind Association should themselves be visually handicapped and the philosophy that blind people must be active participants in the work of the Executive Council and Committees continues to be enshrined in the Royal Charter which now governs the practices of RNIB. Armitage also had a strong belief in the importance of music as a professional pursuit for some blind people and its efficacy for the cultural advancement and leisure activity of others. He urged the provision of greater opportunities for blind people to become trained for the practice of massage and the development of educational practices geared to vocational goals achievable by those without sight, one such avenue of potential employment being piano tuning.

When Francis Campbell came to England in 1868 at the end of a European tour which he had undertaken both to recuperate from an illness and to observe developments at European schools for the blind, he had a fateful meeting with Dr Armitage who was then immersed in the early work of the British and Foreign Blind Association. Campbell, a native of Tennessee, had been blinded as a result of an accident when a small boy, had been educated at the Tennessee School for the Blind where he had developed a passionate interest, and considerable skill, in the performance of music and had taught for short spells at the Tennessee and Wisconsin Schools for the Blind and had for seven years been Head of the Music Department at the famous Perkins School for the Blind in Boston, Massachusetts, under the distinguished Dr Samuel Gridley Howe.

From the very first it was clear that the respective views of Armitage and Campbell concerning the pattern of education for blind youngsters, the importance of music, the relationship between school instruction and employment objectives, were totally compatible and Armitage was quickly able to persuade his new American friend that in Britain lay the opportunity for Campbell to launch the kind of educational programme for the visually handicapped which was so clearly etched in his mind. Money was needed if such an experiment were to be successfully launched and Armitage donated a substantial portion of the required fund and successfully approached some of his wealthy friends to put up the balance. He and Campbell worked together to outline the plan, secure premises, interview potential pupils and their parents, install musical instruments and equipment and publicize the project.

In 1872 the Royal Normal College and Academy of Music for the

Blind, with Francis Campbell as its first Headmaster, opened its doors in Norwood, to the South of London, and so was launched the unique experiment in educational practice, linked to vocational outlets for blind people with special emphasis on music and its associated crafts, which was to become of such tremendous significance to the blind people of Britain and to serve as an example which made a massive impact in Europe and elsewhere. Now known as the Royal National College for the Blind and located in Hereford, the College is a tremendous and still growing force for good, maintaining the highest standards in the provision it makes for the instruction of young blind people in music, piano tuning and repair, commercial and general subjects. For his outstanding service to blind people in Britain, Campbell was knighted by King Edward VII in 1909 and died in 1914, the year which saw the outbreak of the First World War and the blinding of so many young men in battle.

Dr Armitage's labours on behalf of blind youths and adults lasted for thirty years and to his untiring efforts can be traced the creation, in many lands, of new and better training services and heightened levels of professionalism by those who served the blind. He was ever conscious of the responsibility that should be borne by Governments and, with help from the Duke of Westminister, planned a conference which was held in Britain in 1884 which led to the establishment of a Royal Commission to study the conditions of the blind in Great Britain. This inquiry led in turn to the passage in 1893 of the Elementary Education Act which made compulsory the education of all blind children between the ages of six and sixteen. Dr Armitage was to be denied the satisfaction of witnessing the introduction of that particular piece of legislation for which he had worked so diligently, as, during a visit to Ireland in 1890, he was severely injured when thrown from his horse and died within a few days. So ended the life of a man who had triumphed so gallantly over his own blindness and had subsequently worked so diligently and so well to usher in a new era of opportunity for his blind colleagues the world over. His influence goes on today in the work of the Royal National Institute for the Blind whose Executive Council, including many of the blind leaders of today, meet in the Hall which is dedicated to the memory and bears the name of Thomas Rhodes Armitage.

Blindness and visual handicap: the facts

Sir Arthur Pearson

Two years before Dr Armitage founded the British and Foreign Blind Association, which was to develop into the National Institute and subsequently the Royal National Institute for the Blind, there was born in England a child who in later years was to develop into one of the most dynamic personalities of the age and whose adult life would encompass two separate careers, in each of which he left an indelible mark.

Born in 1866, the son of a country parson, the boy who was to become Sir Arthur Pearson early displayed a far-reaching and imaginative mind and a descriptive writing style and it was not surprising that he was attracted to the field of journalism. Upon entering Fleet Street it quickly became apparent to Pearson and his professional colleagues that he had truly found his métier and he climbed rapidly up the journalistic ladder. While still in this thirties he had already become one of the world's great newspaper barons, controlling a string of Britain's most successful national and local dailies and weeklies. His dynamic business and organizational skills were made available to a number of worthy causes and his services to the nation had already secured him a knighthood when in 1910 his sight began to fail, leading to his total blindness two years later.

Pearson was not the type of man to allow loss of sight to consign him to the wings. He had occupied the centre of the stage in one important sphere and he could do so in another. Having through his own sight-loss made contact with the voluntary organizations which were then active in the service of the blind. he recognized that much remained to be accomplished and resolved to lend his best efforts to improve the situation. He became the first President of the National Institute for the Blind, which was then in acute financial difficulty having insufficient resources to complete the building it was erecting in London to serve as its national headquarters. Pearson's unmatched flair for publicity and fund-raising rapidly redeemed the situation and by 1914 the building had been completed and officially opened by His Majesty King George V.

Later that year Europe was plunged into war and Pearson joined with his NIB colleagues in a resolve to ensure that all possible assistance would be extended to those servicemen who would inevitably become blinded on the battlefields. Before long it became sadly apparent that the toll of war blindness would be far greater than could possibly have been anticipated and, although Pearson continued to serve as President of NIB from 1915 to the end of his life, he devoted almost all of his energies to the development of a new organization for the re-training, re-settlement, relief and after-care of blinded soldiers, sailors, and airmen.

Thus was St. Dunstans launched under the personal direction of Sir Arthur Pearson, an organization which has been the world's greatest pioneer in the development and provision of rehabilitation services for the war-blinded. Then, as now, its work bears the imprint of Sir Arthur Pearson's dynamic personality and far-sightedness.

It was always Pearson's philosophy that when people — and particularly those blinded when young — lose their sight they should as rapidly as possible receive the help and training that will enable them to resume every feasible activity of normal life and to help achieve this for the British war blind, he persuaded the Service Chiefs to streamline the referral to St. Dunstans of the blinded casualties. These were received at a fifteen-acre site in Regent's Park in Central London where the adjustment programme began, quickly to be followed by instruction in braille, handicrafts, and occupations.

Always the selection of careers was approached on a personal basis, taking into account the individual's educational and occupational background, skills, aptitudes, and aspirations. Many were helped to enter or return to professional fields while for others a range of vocational training courses were available, enabling them to be employed as masseurs, shorthand typists, telephone switchboard operators, poultry farmers, carpenters and joiners, mat or basket makers, boot and shoe repairers. A staff of resettlement officers made arrangements for them to be placed in jobs, or to set up in business on their own account. When they returned to civilian life they were prepared not only to work but had been restored to a state of fitness in mind and body which enabled them to continue many of the other activities in which they had engaged at St. Dunstans.

All forms of sport were encouraged and it was a common sight for residents of the Regent's Park area to observe blinded servicemen engaging in sprints and long distance running, walking races round the

Outer Circle of the Park, swimming and rowing on the lake. Never in history had young men blinded in battle been provided with such a complete range of supportive services immediately following the onset of blindness and the knowledge that a helping hand would be there to assist with any difficulties that might arise for the rest of their lives.

The St. Dunstans pattern has been duplicated in Commonwealth countries and other lands and the spirit of Sir Arthur Pearson still motivates the work. New heights of achievement were gained in the last war and still today men and women who lose their sight in the service of the Crown, in Northern Ireland or elsewhere, may turn with confidence to St Dunstans for the encouragement, training, and lifelong support that will enable them to rebuild their lives.

Sir Arthur Pearson, the brilliant man of action whose dream of hope for war blinded men and women achieved reality, died in 1921 following an accident in his bath where he fell and struck his head.

Helen Keller

The name of Helen Keller will live for ever and the story of her victorious battle to surmount the most grievous sensory deprivations, is one of the world's greatest sagas of indomitability and accomplishment. Born in Tuscumbia, Alabama, USA, on 27 June 1880, the daughter of a small town newspaper editor who had fought in the Southern Army during the American Civil War, Helen enjoyed a normal babyhood but when only nineteen months old was afflicted with a violent fever which resulted in the loss of sight, hearing, and speech.

When all efforts at cure had failed, Helen's parents sought far and wide for help in rearing and educating the child who, strong and healthy except for her sensory deprivations, was subject to almost uncontrollable temper tantrums, often having to be physically restrained. Their enquiries led them to Dr Anagnos, then Headmaster of Perkins School for the Blind, where some years earlier an encouraging level of success had been recorded in the education of a deaf-blind girl named Laura Bridgman. Dr Anagnos, like his distinguished predecessor, Dr Samuel Gridley Howe, firmly believed that it was possible to pierce the darkness and silence imposed by loss of sight and hearing, to reach the mind of a deaf-blind child and he agreed to send a young partially sighted teacher from his staff to join the Keller household and to work with the afflicted child.

This was Ann Sullivan, the daughter of poor Irish immigrants, who had spent much of her childhood in the workhouse but had overcome poverty, ignorance, and visual loss with indomitable courage. So began the association between Helen and teacher that was to stir the imagination of the whole world. The story of Anne's love for, and struggles with her young charge, how with total lack of response she tapped word after word into the palm of the deaf-blind child using the manual alphabet that had been devised for Laura Bridgman, how enlightenment flooded Helen's mind by the well as Ann tapped out the word 'water' into her palm and how Helen went on to achieve immortality, has been recounted so often in print, on stage, and in film, by radio and television, that it need not be repeated in detail here, but it provides infinitely moving substantiation of the belief that mankind is endowed with innate abilities which, if only they can be tapped, can lead to feats of unbounded accomplishment.

With her teacher ever by her side, Helen quickly learnt to read braille and through this medium as well as the tapping fingers of Anne her mind soaked up education like a sponge. Together they travelled to Boston to be close to the Schools for the Blind and the Deaf. Helen gained admission to the prestigious Radcliffe College the Women's Division of Harvard University, and in 1904 at the age of 24 graduated with an Honours Degree, the first deaf-blind person in history to do so.

This miracle child of Tuscumbia had already become something of a celebrity having been referred to by Mark Twain as one of the most interesting personalities of the nineteenth century and when her first book *The story of my life* was published, first in serial form in the *Ladies Home Journal* and later in hardback, she began to emerge as a world figure. A supremely talented author, her first and subsequent works have been republished in many editions and have an inspirational quality seldom found in other authors. Unfettered by her disabilities, Helen led a most active life, an early worker for women's suffrage and other political causes, a stage performer on America's vaudeville circuit she was one of history's great champions for the education and rehabilitation of handicapped people, particularly those who were blind or deaf.

Blindness and visual handicap: the facts

Although she laboured constantly to achieve complete clarity of speech, this was never totally accomplished. Yet she crossed and recrossed the United States attending meetings, addressing State legislatures, visiting the Halls of Congress in Washington and achieving the enactment of State and Federal Laws that served as the basis of the all-embracing programmes for the handicapped which exist today.

During the Great War she learnt of the work of St. Dunstans and with an American business man, George Kessler, who had survived the sinking of the *Lusitania* she helped to found an American organization to assist with the rehabilitation of blinded servicemen of all the Allied Armies. This organization was later to become the American Foundation for Overseas Blind, more recently renamed Helen Keller International and its world-wide activities have fostered the development of adequate programmes for blind people in every continent on earth.

In 1921 she joined with Major M. C. Migel to establish the American Foundation for the Blind which has for the past sixty years served as one of the world's great authorities on every aspect of service to the blind and the deaf-blind, having had a most powerful voice in the development throughout the United States of a chain of Local, State, and Federal services and a network of voluntary organizations for the blind and the deaf-blind that is unsurpassed in the world. Helen Keller, who following the death of her beloved friend and mentor Anne Sullivan in 1936 had recruited the Scottish born Polly Thomson as her companion, continued to serve as national and international counsellor to the American Foundation for the Blind and the American Foundation for Overseas Blind until the day of her death.

In her later years Helen devoted the greater part of her working life to the provision of assistance to the blind in the many countries of the world who recognized her as their inspiring leader. Tirelessly she travelled across the entire globe, seeking out and pleading the cause of her blind comrades everywhere and the success of her missionary endeavours can be seen in the programmes that developed as a direct result of her personal intervention. Schools and centres bearing her name can be found in every part of the world and no full accounting can ever be made of the impact her work brought to bear on the lives of blind and deaf-blind men, women and children everywhere.

Helen Keller died at her home in Westport, Connecticut, shortly before reaching her 88th birthday in June 1968 following a lengthy illness. At the memorial service held in the Washington National Cathedral, the great and lowly people of the world, including contingents of blind, of deaf, and of deaf-blind people, gathered to pay homage to the gallant woman, who, more than any other person of the twentieth century, had brought accelerated impetus to the provision of programmes for the enlightenment, education, training, and general welfare of all who must live their lives hampered by serious sensory deprivation.

And so the work for the blind goes on having been passed from hand to hand by the pioneers of the past to those who function in the present day. The spirit of progress still motivates the work which now circles the globe and powerful international organizations, including the United Nations, play their full part in achieving a pace of progress that bodes well for the future. Blind people, both as individuals and through their local national and international organizations, are playing an ever increasing part towards their own advancement, giving ever greater strength to the partnership between the sighted and the sightless, which has contributed so much throughout the years.

25

International co-operation

With the establishment and growth throughout the nineteenth and early twentieth centuries of educational programmes for blind children and services for the training, employment, and general welfare of blind adults, came an increasing need for those who were responsible for conducting such activities in their own countries to keep abreast of developments that were occurring elsewhere and to exchange experiences and discuss common problems for the more rapid and effective progress of blind welfare services everywhere. Such exchanges reached a crescendo in the late nineteenth century and the early years of this century, as the proponents of the braille code and those who supported alternative methods of producing embossed print for the blind waged what was to come to be known as 'The battle of the dots'. Impetus was given to international exchanges and joint planning by the large numbers of blind created by the Great War of 1914–18.

The World Council for the Welfare of the Blind became a legal entity at an Assembly in Paris in July 1951. Membership is open to any country and the delgations are composed of representatives of organizations of or for the blind. This brought to fruition work commenced in New York twenty years earlier.

International non-governmental organizations

The establishment of the World Council for the Welfare of the Blind was the first of a series of international non-governmental organizations, each of which, in its own particular sphere of interest has made a substantial contribution for the benefit of blind people, and whose influence on governmental thought and action has been of great significance. Four such organizations, which co-operate closely, discharge particularly important functions and their roles are briefly discussed.

International co-operation

World Council for the Welfare of the Blind

World Assemblies occur at intervals of not more than five years. More than 70 countries are now full members of the Council and appropriate organizations and individuals serve as international, sponsoring, or associate members. Certain individuals who have contributed outstandingly to the creation or development of activities of great value to blind people may be elected by the World Assembly to honorary life membership. Between meetings of the General Assembly, the affairs of the Council are conducted by an executive committee whose members are elected on a regional basis. Regional committees, which bring together the elected representatives of organizations of and for the blind in different areas of the world now exist in Europe, the Middle East, Africa, Asia, Latin America, and North America-Oceania. Each of these regional committees meets regularly and several have established subcommittees or commissions which are responsible for conducting in-depth studies on specific professional topics in a regional rather than a world context.

At the international level, standing committees are active in a number of special-interest areas including the prevention of blindness, finance, social development, cultural affairs, development co-operation, services to the deaf-blind, rehabilitation training and employment, sporting and recreational activities. The World Council for the Welfare of the Blind has a consultative relationship with the United Nations and all of its relevant specialized agencies, including UNESCO, UNICEF, ILO, and WHO. It is a founder-member of the Council of World Organizations Interested in the Handicapped and has established close working relationships with many other international organizations whose activities impinge on the lives and activities of people who are blind.

International Council for the Education of the Visually Handicapped

This organization is concerned with the special needs of blind children. In addition to the meetings of the General Assembly and the regional bodies, special conferences are frequently arranged to study specific aspects of the education of young blind people, for example, educational techniques; the provision of instruction in specific subjects; the

211

problems peculiar to the education of certain special groups such as pre-school children, the deaf-blind, or visually handicapped children with additional physical disabilities; the integration of blind children in ordinary schools, and the special problems of the developing world.

Under the auspices of the International Council for the Education of the Visually Handicapped or its regional committees teacher exchanges are arranged and teams of experts are assembled to visit and give intensive courses of instruction to teachers in countries wishing to establish new schools or improve existing services. Aid is also provided to developing countries by the collection and shipment of substantial quantities of special teaching aids, apparatus and braille books.

The International Council for the Education of the Visually Handicapped enjoys consultative relationships with UNESCO and UNICEF, and has been instrumental in encouraging these organizations to give special emphasis in their programmes to the special needs of blind children, particularly through the assignment of consultants, allocation of fellowships and scholarships,and by encouraging member nations to expand and modernize their educational programmes for visually handicapped youth.

International Federation of the Blind

In 1964 a group of thirteen blind people, six from the United States and seven from countries of the developing world founded this international body. In 1980 the number of affiliated countries was 62. There are three regional committees in Europe, Africa, and Asia. Only organized movements of blind people may become full members of The International Federation of the Blind, but other organizations may apply for associate membership. The aim of the International Federation of the Blind is to serve 'the blind of all nations, operated by the blind of all nations for the blind of all nations' and 'to provide a forum for collective self expression and discussion by the blind of the world and to act as the articulate voice for their joint discussions and common objectives'.

As the constitutions both of World Council for the Welfare of the Blind and the International Federation of the Blind recognize the right of blind people to participate actively in the conduct of national and international activities undertaken on their behalf, a high level of co-operation between the two international bodies has developed in recent years.

The International Federation of the Blind enjoys a consultative relationship with the United Nations and its specialized agencies.

International Agency for the Prevention of Blindness

Since its establishment in January 1975, the membership of the International Agency for the Prevention of Blindness has grown rapidly and the Agency has had excellent initial results in its aim of eradication throughout the world of many of the avoidable diseases and conditions which cause blindness. The organization, which is composed of experts from the fields of medicine, nutrition, and other related disciplines as well as organizations of and for the blind, works in close co-operation with United Nations bodies, particularly WHO and UNICEF, and has enlisted the support of bodies such as the World Bank to launch comprehensive programmes aimed to make substantial inroads into the incidence of unnecessary blindness, particularly in developing countries, before the end of the century.

As a result of the support of the International Agency for the Prevention of Blindness, national committees have now been established throughout the world. Such committees are composed of distinguished administrators and practitioners in general fields of medicine, ophthalmology, nutrition, and eye research, together with representatives of national organizations of and for the blind. They evaluate requests for financial support, for the introduction or extension of projects in the field of ophthalmic research in universities and hospital departments, and allocate funds for broad programmes of blindness prevention in the developing world. In addition to conducting such programmes on their own account, many national committees allocate a proportion of their annual income to the International Agency.

A large proportion of the estimated 42 million people of the world who fall within the generally accepted definition of blindness have lost their sight as a result of the onset of trachoma, onchocerciasis (sometimes known as 'river blindness'), cataracts, or nutritional blindness resulting from vitamin A deficiency. The International Agency for the

213

Blindness and visual handicap: the facts

Prevention of Blindness and its national affiliates are now harnessing massive aid for the worldwide attack on these scourges. The incidence of trachoma has been dramatically reduced through the introduction of improved hygiene and the cure of existing cases with antibiotic ointment. Onchocerciasis, which has caused blindness among up to 30 per cent of village populations of some areas of West Africa and Central America, is transmitted by a fly which breeds in pools on river banks, and spectacular results are being achieved by international action to eradicate the pest. The surgical removal of cataracts is now being undertaken on a massive scale in many parts of Asia and Africa, through the formation of mobile teams of ophthalmologists and auxiliaries who set up temporary eye camps, where a hundred or more successful operations may be performed in a single day. Nutritional blindness is being attacked on a broad scale in many countries through the organization of teams who undertake the mass distribution of vitamin A tablets or capsules and instruct local nurses and village leaders concerning dosage and the establishment of local distribution centres. Instruction at regional and sub-regional centres is designed to change long-established dietary habits which often make no use of green vegetables, the lack of which can lead rapidly to blindness among newly weaned babies and young children.

International aid

It is now possible for countries in need to benefit from a growing programme of international aid. The division of social affairs of the United Nations, and many of UN's specialized agencies, are able to allocate the long- or short-term services of special consultants, set up demonstration projects, organize staff training courses, arrange overseas travel fellowships and scholarships, donate specialized equipment, and assist requesting countries in a variety of other ways.

A number of international non-governmental organizations also maintain programmes for the provision of assistance to services for the blind, among these are the World Council for the Welfare of the Blind and the International Federation of the Blind. Several important organizations are nationally based but exist solely to assist the development of programmes for the blind and the prevention of blindness in

214

other countries. The Royal Commonwealth Society for the Blind maintains an extensive programme of assistance to governments and to non-governmental programmes for the visually handicapped in all those Commonwealth countries which are in need of such support. Helen Keller International (formerly the American Foundation for Overseas Blind), which was originally established to initiate special programmes for the rehabilitation of men blinded in battle during the First World War, now maintains a worldwide operation covering all aspects of education, rehabilitation, training employment, and welfare of visually handicapped men, women, and children, regardless of the cause of their disability. In addition, Helen Keller International has initiated numerous projects in countries where the incidence of controllable eye ailments is unacceptably high. A similar organization based in the Federal Republic of Germany, Christoffel-Blindenmission helps those concerned with the creation and improvement of blind welfare activity, particularly in the developing countries. Each of these three organizations has overseas representatives responsible for maintaining local contacts and providing advice and guidance in the supervision of current projects.

Voluntary organizations for the blind in a number of countries provide personnel, equipment, and study grants, and organize conferences, sometimes merging their efforts to set up multilateral aid programmes for the more rapid progress of their development programmes.

26

How can we help?

Many people would like to help their blind neighbours to surmount some of their difficulties and thus to lead fuller, more interesting, and more rewarding lives. Yet many who are so motivated are totally unfamiliar with the subject of blindness and the difficulties it can generate so that a chance encounter with a blind person too frequently proves to be an embarrassing experience for both parties, unlikely to develop into a constructive relationship from which something of permanent value will emerge.

The ways in which volunteer help can be used in the service of blind people are legion and some of them will be mentioned in this chapter. But many readers will simply wish to know how they can give a helping hand to the blind man or woman they may meet casually in the street; what sort of action they might take to lighten the load of a blind neighbour; or whether, in fact, such help might be welcomed. There is no simple answer to questions such as these, as the type of assistance that will be of most value and therefore received most gratefully will depend entirely on the circumstances of the moment.

It is important not to have a stereotypic image of 'the typical blind person', for there is no such thing. People who are without sight are just as varied in terms of disposition, level of intelligence, range of interests, sense of humour — or lack of it —, courtesy, political or religious beliefs and so on, as any other cross-section of society. Thus, the key to a positive relationship, be it of the briefest kind, will be simply to recognize that one is dealing with an ordinary person who cannot see, and not a member of a race apart.

In the street

Help is best given quietly and without fuss. Generally speaking, the blind hate to be a nuisance to others and dislike having public attention drawn to their disabilities and their difficulties. The self appointed aide who precedes a blind traveller along the pavement demanding all and sundry to 'stand aside — here comes a blind man' is serving only to embarrass the blind person he seeks to help. If he is striding out confidently with a cane and maintaining a straight course the blind person probably needs no particular help. If he appears to falter or lack decisiveness in his actions, particularly if a road crossing or other danger-point is being approached, the simple question: 'Can I help in any way?' will usually bring a quick and grateful response.

If called upon to guide a blind person across the street, or on a longer journey, allow him to take your arm, slightly above the elbow, and proceed at a normal pace, with your blind companion walking half a step behind. This will permit him to detect and compensate for changes of direction. Pause very briefly before stepping down or up kerbs and, particularly if he is taller than you, remember to keep an eye open to warn him about overhead hazards such as overhanging branches or shop blinds.

In the home or neighbourhood

Most blind people have normal hearing, so that conversations in the street or the home should be conducted in a normal voice. Avoid expressing sympathy in over extravagant terms. If you have a blind neighbour who you know to be living alone, particularly if he or she is elderly, it would be a kindly act to visit the home, to introduce yourself, and let it be known that you are willing to help with difficulties that may arise. If such an initial approach is made in a friendly, non-gushing way, it will almost certainly evoke a positive response. As the ice is broken, the conversation will enable you to identify the ways in which you can be helpful without unnecessarily intruding upon the private life of the person concerned.

Occasionally you may wish to help a blind person to become seated, for example, in a restaurant, and if this is handled badly, your companion can easily be made to feel that he has become the central figure in something of an exhibition. It is a simple matter for the operation to be handled discreetly. If the blind person is holding your elbow, you may simply place your own hand on the back of the chair, thus enabling him to locate it and then to slip quietly around to take his seat. When leaving, let your companion know that you are standing up and that you will proceed to the back of his chair: he can then rise and take your elbow. These examples are included simply to emphasize the fact that ordinary acts of helpfulness can be conducted without fuss and bother, and if this is done your blind friend will be doubly appreciative.

If included among guests at your home or in a group elsewhere, try to ensure that the blind individual neither becomes the central focus of the conversation nor is excluded from it. In brief, act naturally and allow him to do so. Normally the fact that he is blind need never come up in the conversation; but if it does, try not to allow the subject to become over-dramatized; most blind people have at some time been posed the inane and unanswerable question: 'What is it like to be blind?', and they tend to resent that: as they do the assertion: 'I think you are marvellous if I were blind I think I would kill myself!'

During conversation in a group which includes a blind person, try to remember that he lacks the visual evidence which would enable him to determine whether you are addressing him or some other person in the room. A question such as: 'What do you think about that?' may leave him wondering whether he is expected to respond, or whether the question was directed elsewhere: add his name so he is left in no doubt. Simple little tricks such as these can be of vital importance in putting a visually handicapped individual at ease and can convert a stilted conversation into an easy and friendly exchange.

Local and national organizations for the blind

Guidance on how your services as a regular or occasional volunteer helper for the blind can best be used can be secured by contacting the nearest state or voluntary agency for the blind. Such associations exist in most of the larger cities, and maintain varied programmes. Many of the blind people they serve may be elderly and lonely and your offer to become a new and helpful friend to some such individual would be welcomed gladly.

Many of the local agencies as well as some state and national bodies operate residential homes, particularly for the elderly blind; hostels for blind people in work; and holiday homes and hotels for summer or year-round visually handicapped visitors. Volunteers can help by organizing or joining in recreational activities, accompanying blind residents on shopping expeditions, reading letters and so on. In this way they add substantially to the effectiveness of the work and the content-ment of the blind residents, and your help will be eagerly channelled to where it could be of maximum advantage.

If you are a car-owner and would be willing to help transport visually handicapped men and women, possibly including some with additional physical handicaps, to and from weekly club meetings, for example, your local governmental or private agency will welcome you with open arms, as will the blind beneficiaries of your kindness.

Braille and recorded material

Many blind people, particularly those engaged in levels of higher and further education need textbooks and other material in braille or recor-ded form. In order to satisfy this need most countries maintain student braille and tape libraries, much of the material for which is produced by volunteers working in their own homes either independently, or as members of local groups. Special skills are required by volunteer braill-ists, and those who wish to become proficient but who have little or no knowledge of the system can take a correspondence course leading to a certificate enabling them to undertake work for the student braille library or one of the local groups.

Those wishing to undertake volunteer recording work should own standard tape recorders, have pleasant voices which reproduce well, and be able to present in a comprehensible and professional manner the sometimes technical material they are called upon to read. They are usually expected to devote at least a couple of hours a day to the task.

The United States Library of Congress in Washington, DC is com-pletely funded from Federal government sources and through its National Library Service for the Blind and Physically Handicapped maintains the world's largest programme for the provision of reading material of all kinds on loan to blind people. Distribution of books in braille and recorded form is effected through its 56 regional libraries. As part of its programme the Library of Congress utilizes the service of volunteer braillists for the production of hand-transcribed books and works in close co-operation with the National Braille Association which co-ordinates the activities of many volunteer groups throughout the country. Information can be obtained from either of these sources about the availability of braille instruction courses by mail. Trained and potential volunteer transcribers can be put in touch with local transcribing groups and with organizations, schools, and students to whom help could be extended. Those who may be willing to tape-record books for blind students may also approach the National Library Service for the Blind and Physically Handicapped of the Library of Congress for information on that subject or Recording for the Blind Inc under whose auspices volunteer recording groups are active at locations throughout the country.

In the United Kingdom the Royal National Institute for the Blind maintains the most extensive student braille and tape libraries for which most of the books are produced by volunteers. The RNIB offers a course of instruction by post to all who wish to become proficient in braille for the purpose of offering their services to the student braille library or to one of the several local groups which produce textbooks for blind students at universities in their localities or meet the direct needs of individuals. Those who may wish to volunteer their service as tape recordists and who possess tape recording machines should approach the RNIB indicating the subjects in which they feel qualified to serve as readers. A voice test will then be arranged prior to admission to the scheme.

In Australia most of the state institutes and schools for the blind offer supportive services to visually handicapped people attending universities and specialized courses of further education. Such assistance includes the provision of braille and tape material much of which is produced by volunteers. Those willing to serve the blind in such ways should approach their state institutes to obtain full information about current training opportunities and details of required qualifications. Residents of New Zealand seeking similar guidance may contact the National Headquarters or any of the regional offices of the Royal New Zealand Foundation for the Blind while the national headquarters of the Canadian National Institute for the Blind or any of its provincial offices will welcome an approach from any potential volunteer braillist or recordist willing to be of direct assistance to blind people in that country. The School for the Blind at Worcester is South Africa's oldest and one of the most active organizations providing help to blind people at all levels of education including those attending universities. Volunteers are used for the production of braille and recorded literature and the School will be pleased to offer advice and assistance as will any of the state or local organizations for the blind which are affiliated to the South African National Council for the Blind.

Escort service

Blind people are now doing more national and international travelling than in the past. Lengthy and unfamiliar journeys, particularly those which may involve changes between termini, pose serious difficulties. In most countries national, state, or local agencies for the blind have established formal or informal escort services which are staffed by volunteers. A blind man or woman arriving from abroad can be met at the airport and accompanied, either by car or public transport, to his hotel, or to a railway station. A similar service is available to blind people travelling by train or coach within the country concerned. If you would be prepared to be on call to provide such a service from time to time your local agency for the blind would be delighted to hear from you.

Talking Newspapers

In an increasing number of areas throughout the world, volunteer groups have been established to record for the benefit of blind people items drawn from national or local newspapers. A wide variety of skills are required of the volunteers, who select and edit appropriate items from local newspapers, maintain lists of members and their addresses, place recorded cassettes in postal containers; type and insert address labels; post, deliver or repair play-back machines, and take part, either as engineers or presenters, at the recording sessions, which usually occur weekly.

The Talking Newspaper Service performs a vital function in the integration of blind people in their communities, and those who are able to devote a reasonable amount of time on a regular basis are giving valuable help. If you are drawn to this form of volunteer activity you

221

should contact your local Talking Newspaper. Full details are obtainable from the local office of your national agency for the blind. In the United States programmes of this kind are co-ordinated by Recordings for the Blind Inc, and in Britain by the Talking Newspaper Association of UK.

Sharing special interests

Many blind people wish to continue their special interests or hobbies after the onset of blindness; these can often be maintained without serious difficulty. It gives particular satisfaction to the blind person if he can pursue such interests in the company of sighted friends rather than in a segregated setting. This usually involves members of special interest groups giving a little thought to and perhaps considering minor modifications of their activities. Examples of such programmes are: music circles, dramatic and operatic societies, bridge and whist clubs (where the blind player would be permitted to use braille playing cards), discussion groups, debating societies, Women's Institutes, Towns-women's Guilds, men's clubs, and church activities of all kinds.

The programmes of some special interest groups may not lend them-selves to the full participation of blind members. Nevertheless, the organizations and their individual participants may have talents or areas of special knowledge from which much enjoyment and instruction could be gained by people whose blindness precludes their direct invol-vement.

The lives of residents in special homes or hostels for the blind can be greatly enlivened by visits from choirs, soloists, drama groups, and speakers. Organizations which conduct clubs for the visually handi-capped are frequently hard-pressed to arrange varied and interesting programmes for the club season, and would be most grateful if you could offer to arrange an evening of interest and entertainment.

Cornea donation

Many people become blind as a result of ulceration or other damage to the cornea, the transparent outer layer of the eye covering the pupil, and it is frequently possible for sight to be restored through the transplantation of new corneae. These are obtained by removing the eyes very soon after the death of individuals who during their lifetime have entered into the necessary agreement. In some instances the next-of-kin of a person who has died in hospital and who may not have entered into an eye-donor agreement is approached by the hospital authorities for permission to remove the eyes to restore sight to another patient who is urgently awaiting a corneal transplant operation. When a registered donor dies, arrangements should immediately be made with the hospital or doctor for the eyes to be excised and sent to the Eye Bank, where the corneae will be tissue-typed prior to transplantation to an appropriate recipient.

Corneal transplantation has restored sight to many thousands of blind people. If any reader of any age would like to make such a bequest, his family doctor or the Ophthalmic Department of his local hospital should be approached for full information. It is not the practice to remove an eye from a living donor to transplant to a relative, friend, or other individual.

Donations and legacies

Blind welfare services in most countries are largely maintained through the activities of national, regional, and local societies for the blind, who are dependent upon charitable contributions for the maintenance and extension of their services. The increasing expense of such services, particularly since the development of costly technological equipment, has placed a great strain on the resources of most voluntary bodies. Only if the generosity of the general public, of charitable foundations, professional and business organizations and research bodies is maintained will the visually handicapped continue to receive all the help they need. When preparing their wills, individuals may wish to consider naming one of the national or local agencies for the blind as the recipient of a specific bequest or as a residuary legatee.

Some may also wish to assist charitable organizations for the blind in their fund-raising campaigns and efforts. Much of the work entailed in such fund-raising activities is undertaken by volunteers who serve as house-to-house or street collectors on flag days, organize coffee mornings, 'bring and buy' sales, sponsored walks and other such events, and a host of other methods of securing donations from friends, the general public and organizations. There is an ever-growing need for volunteers willing to devote even a small amount of time to such work, and potential helpers should get in touch with their national or local voluntary agency for the blind.

Careers in work for the blind

The principal purpose of this chapter has been to identify some of the ways in which people give of their time and talents as voluntary workers for the blind. However, some of our readers may be interested in a career in blind welfare. This can be very rewarding, and those who enter the field usually find the work so personally stimulating and absorbing that they seldom regret their choice of career. Openings exist from time to time on the staffs of national, regional, and local agencies for the blind; rehabilitation and training centres; libraries; secondary, primary, and nursery schools; homes, hostels, and hotels; braille and Moon printing works. Individuals with a wide range of skills and interests may hope to find such employment which is suited to their talents and past experience, while gaining additional satisfaction from the knowledge that they are helping those in need.

All organizations that extend services to the blind try to ensure that the highest professional levels are maintained. Their staff must be fully qualified by education, training, or experience. Those who wish to become rehabilitation teachers, Technical Officers, or social workers for the blind should have secured an appropriate university degree or a nationally recognized diploma. Orientation and Mobility Officers need special training and courses are offered by some universities or at centres conducted by national organizations for the blind.

Animal lovers may be attracted to careers as dog-handlers and instructors for blind people being trained with their guide dogs. All accredited guide dog agencies can supply details of necessary qualifications.

All those wishing to provide educational services to visually handicapped children must be fully qualified teachers and have obtained or be willing to secure a further diploma covering the special techniques of educating blind children. In the United States, United Kingdom, and some other countries special diploma courses are available at selected universities, but elsewhere the training is undertaken at schools for the blind or by correspondence.

Those interested in a career as a house mother or father or other post on the child care staff of residential schools and nursery units for blind children should obtain appropriate qualifications. A full-time in-service training course is maintained at some schools, as well as within residential homes, hostels, and holiday hotels, positions ranging from managers and wardens to cooks, kitchen staff, and cleaners are also available. Individuals with special abilities and qualifications in particular professions, skills, and crafts can join the staff of rehabilitation and training centres, workshops for the blind, or within a local home workers scheme.

Computers are being increasingly used in the special services for the blind, including the production of braille books, the operation of library and other services, and in accountancy, and people with experience as data analysts and key punchers are needed in a number of blind welfare settings, as are those with clerical, secretarial, and other office skills.

Countless opportunities exist for individuals to help blind men, women, and children, either as volunteers or as paid employees. We hope that many who read this will respond to the challenge and, to those who do, we extend warmest thanks and our wishes for happiness and success in their chosen field of endeavour.

Further reading

Part I

Hogan, M. J. and Zimmerman, L. E. (1962). *Ophthalmic pathology.* W. B. Saunders Company, Philadelphia.

Duke Elder, W. S. and Perkins, E. S. (1966). Diseases of the uveal tract. *System of ophthalmology* Vol. IX. Kimpton, London.

Duke Elder, W. S. and Dobree, J. H. (1967). Diseases of the retina. *System of ophthalmology* Vol. X. Kimpton, London.

Wilson, J. (1980). *World blindness and its prevention.* Oxford University Press.

Michaelson, I. C. and Berman, E. R. (1972). *Causes and prevention of Blindness.* Academic Press, New York.

Roper-Hall, M. J. (1980). *Stallard's eye surgery*, 6th edn. Wright, Bristol.

Davson, H. (1980). *Physiology of the eye*, (4th edn). Churchill Livingstone, Edinburgh.

Clifford Rose, F. (1976). *Medical ophthalmology*, C. V. Mosby Company, St. Louis.

HMSO (1979). *Blindness and partial sight in England* 1969–76 DHSS Report No. 129, HMSO, London.

Jopling, W. H. (1978). *Handbook of leprosy* (2nd edn). Heinemann, London.

Michaelson, I. C. (1980). *Text-book of the diseases of the fundus of the eye* (3rd edn). Churchill Livingstone, Edinburgh.

Part II

Carroll, T. J. (1961). *Blindness: what it is, what it does and how to live with it.* Little, Brown and Co., Boston.

Chapman, E. K. (1978). *Visually handicapped children and young people.* Routledge & Kegan Paul, London.

Cutsforth, T. D. (1951). *The blind in school and society: a psychological study* (revised edn). American Foundation for the Blind, New York.

Department of Education and Science (1972). *The education of the visually handicapped.* Report of the Committee of Enquiry appointed by the Secretary of State for Education and Science in October, 1968. HMSO, London.

Ford, F. and Heshel, T. (1977). *In touch: aids and services for blind and partially sighted people* (revised edn). British Broadcasting Corporation, London.

Freeman, P. (1975). *Understanding the deaf/blind child.* Heinemann, London.

Guide Dogs for the Blind Association (1981). *Fifty years forward: the story of guide dogs in Britain.* GDBA, Windsor.

Gill, J. and Reid, F. (1975). In *The handicapped person in the community: a post-experience course.* Unit 6: *Visual handicap: aids and support.* Open University Press, Milton Keynes.

International Agency for the Prevention of Blindness (ed. Sir John Wilson). (1980). *World blindness and its prevention.* Oxford University Press.

Jamieson, M., Parlett, M., and Pocklington, K. (1977). *Towards integration: a study of blind and partially sighted children in ordinary schools.* NFER, Windsor.

Klemz, A. (1977). *Blindness and partial sight: a guide for social workers and others concerned with the care and rehabilitation of the visually handicapped.* Woodhead-Faulkner, Cambridge.

Lowenfeld, B. (1975). *The changing status of the blind: from separation to integration.* Charles C. Thomas, Springfield, Ill.

Mackenzie, Sir C. (1954). *World braille usage: a survey of efforts towards uniformity of braille notation.* Unesco, Paris. (New edition in preparation).

Rose, J. (1970). *Changing focus: the development of blind welfare in Britain.* Hutchinson, London.

Ross, I. (1951). *Journey into light: the story of the education of the blind.* Appleton-Century-Crofts, New York.

Royal National Institute for the Blind (1980). *Directory of agencies for the blind in the British Isles and overseas,* (revised edn). RNIB in association with Gardner's Trust for the Blind, London.

Royal National Institute for the Blind. (1979). Report of Working Party on the Employment of Blind People. RNIB, London.

Scott, E. P., Jan, E. and Freeman, D. (1977). *Can't your child see?* University Park Press, Baltimore, MD.

Scott, R. A. (1969). *The making of blind men: a study of adult socialization.* Russell Sage Foundation, New York.

Welsh, R. L. and Blasch, B. B. (eds) (1980). *Foundations of orientation and mobility.* American Foundation for the Blind, New York.

International and national organizations for the blind

International agencies

International Agency for the Prevention of Blindness, Commonwealth House, Haywards Heath, West Sussex, RH16 3AZ, UK.

International Council for Education of the Visually Handicapped, Postfach 364, D–6140 Bensheim 1, Federal Republic of Germany.

International Federation of the Blind, Mastweg 2, B2610 Wilrijk, Belgium.

World Council for the Welfare of the Blind, 58 Avenue Bosquet, 75007 Paris, France.

Organizations maintaining international aid programmes

Christoffel Blindenmission, Nibelungenstrasse 124, D–6140 Bensheim 4, Federal Republic of Germany.

Helen Keller International Inc., 22 West 17 Street, New York, NY 10011, USA.

Royal Commonwealth Society for the Blind, Commonwealth House, Heath Road, Haywards Heath, West Sussex, RH16 3AZ, UK.

Swedish Federation of the Visually Handicapped, S–122 BB, Enskade.

National organizations

Australia

Australian Federation of Blind Citizens, 18 Albert Avenue, Tranmere, S.A. 5073.

Australian National Council for the Blind, 7 Mair Street, Brighton Beach, Victoria 3188.

Bangladesh

Bangladesh National Society for the Blind, 12 Folder Street, Wari, Dacca 3.

Canada

Canadian Council of the Blind, 99 Henderson Street, Riverview, New Brunswick, EIB 4B6.

Canadian National Institute for the Blind, 1929 Bayview Avenue, Toronto, Ontario M4G 3E8.

Ghana

Ghana Society for the Blind, PO Box 3065, Accra.

Hong Kong

Hong Kong Society for the Blind, 33 Granville Road, Kowloon.

India

National Association for the Blind, Jehangir Wadia Building, 51 Mahatma Gandhi Road, Bombay 400 023.

National Institute for the Visually Handicapped, Department of Social Welfare, Government of India, Rajpur Road, Dehra Dun, Uttar Pradesh.

Ireland

National Council for the Blind of Ireland, Armitage House, 10 Lower Hatch Street, Dublin 2.

National League of the Blind of Ireland, 35 Gardiner Place, Dublin 1.

Kenya

Kenya Society for the Blind, PO Box 46656, Nairobi.

Malaysia

Malayan Association for the Blind, PO Box 687, Kuala Lumpur.

New Zealand

New Zealand Association of the Blind and Partially Blind, 3 Lauriston Avenue, Remuera, Auckland 5.

Royal New Zealand Foundation for the Blind, 545 Parnell Road, Private Bag, Newmarket, Auckland 1.

Nigeria

Nigeria National Advisory Council for the Blind, PO Box 2145, 15 Martin Street, Lagos.

Pakistan

Pakistan Association of the Blind, 4 Noor House, P-56 Victoria Road, Karachi 3.

Singapore

Singapore Association for the Blind, 47 Toa Payoh Rise, Singapore 11.

International and national organizations for the blind

South Africa

South African National Council for the Blind, 1st Floor, NOSA Building, 508 Proes Street, Arcadia, Pretoria 0007.

United Kingdom

Association for the Education and Welfare of the Visually Handicapped, East Anglian School, Church Road, Gorleston-on-Sea, Great Yarmouth, Norfolk, NR31 6LP.

British Computer Association of the Blind, BCM Box 950, London WC1.

British National Committee for the Prevention of Blindness, 191 Old Marylebone Road, London NW1 5QN.

Guide Dogs for the Blind Association, Park Street, Windsor, Berks.

National Association for Deaf/Blind and Rubella Handicapped, 164 Cromwell Lane, Coventry, West Midlands, CV4 8AP.

National Association of Orientation and Mobility Instructors, 31 Tennyson Road, Hutton, Brentwood, Essex.

National Association of Technical Officers for the Blind, 34 Panmure Road, London, SE26.

National Federation of the Blind, 45 South Street, Normanton, West Yorkshire, WF6 1EE.

National League of the Blind and Disabled, 2 Tenterden Road, London N17 8BE.

National Library for the Blind, Cromwell Road, Bredbury, Stockport, SK6 2SG.

Partially-Sighted Society, Breaston, Derbyshire DE7 3UE.

Royal National Institute for the Blind, 224 Great Portland Street, London W1N 6AA.

Scottish Braille Press, Craigmillar Park, Edinburgh, Lothian EH16 5NB.

St. Dunstan's Organization for Men and Women Blinded on War Service, PO Box 58, 191 Old Marylebone Road, London NW1 5QN.

Visual Impairment Association, Royal Leicestershire, Rutland and Wycliffe Society for the Blind, Margaret Road, Leicester, LE5 5FU.

USA

Affiliated Leadership League of and for the Blind of America, 879 Park Avenue, Baltimore, Maryland, 21201.

American Association of Workers for the Blind, Inc., 1511 K Street NW, Washington, DC. 20005.

American Council of the Blind, Inc., 1211 Connecticut Avenue, N.W. Suite 506, Washington, DC 20036.

American Foundation for the Blind, Inc., 15 West 16 Street, New York, NY 10011.

American Printing House for the Blind, 1839 Frankfort Avenue, Louisville, Ky. 40206.

Association for Education of the Visually Handicapped, 919 Walnut Street, 7th Floor, Philadelphia, Pa. 19107.

Blinded Veterans Association, 1735 DeSales Street, NW, Washington, DC 20036.

Braille Institute of America, Inc., 741 North Vermont Avenue, Los Angeles, California 90029.

Clovernook Printing House for the Blind, 7000 Hamilton Avenue, Cincinnati, Ohio, 45231.

Eye Bank Association of America, Inc., 6560 Fannin Street, Houston, Texas 77030.

Howe Press of Perkins School for the Blind, 175 North Beacon Street, Watertown, Mass. 02172.

Library of Congress, National Library Service for Blind and Physically Handicapped, 1291 Taylor Street, NW Washington, DC 20542.

National Braille Association, 654A Godwin Avenue, Midland Park, NJ 07432.

National Braille Press, Inc., 88 St. Stephen Street, Boston, Mass. 02115.

National Federation of the Blind, 1800 Johnston Street, Baltimore, Maryland, 21230.

National Industries for the Blind, 1455 Broad Street, Bloomfield, NJ 07003.

National Institutes of Health, National Eye Institute, Bethesda, Maryland, 20205.

National Society for the Prevention of Blindness, 79 Madison Avenue, New York, NY 10016.

Recording for the Blind, Inc., 215 East 58 Street, New York, NY.

The Seeing Eye, Inc., PO Box 375, Morristown, NJ 07960.

Vision Foundation, Inc., 770 Centre Street, Newton, MA 02158.

West Indies

Caribbean Council for the Blind, 118 Duke Street, Port of Spain, Trinidad.

Glossary

adhesion: pathological bonding of tissues.

amblyopia: dimness of vision without detectable organic disease of the eye.

aneurysm: a localized distension of the wall of a blood-vessel.

antibiotic: drug hindering bacterial growth.

antihistamine: anti-allergic drug.

angle of the anterior chamber: the recess formed between the front of the iris and the back of the cornea. Route for escape of intra-ocular fluid.

anterior chamber: space between the cornea and crystalline lens.

arteriosclerosis: hardening of the arteries.

arthritis: inflammation of one or more joints.

aseptic: sterile, without contamination by microorganisms.

blood cells: red cells (erythrocytes), white cells, (leucocytes), and platelets.

capillary (vessels): minute tubes connecting smaller arteries and veins.

cartilage: firm supporting tissue, especially on joint surfaces.

chalazion: miebomian cyst, caused by distension of gland of eyelid.

chromosome: rod shaped bodies in the nuclei of cells containing genes or hereditary factors.

congenital: existing at (and usually before) birth.

connective tissue: supporting framework of body structures composed of collagen.

contusion: bruise.

corticosteroids: see steroids.

cortex (of brain): perceptive outer layers of brain (grey matter)

dendritic: branched like a tree.

diplopia: double vision (two separate images).

dystrophy: degenerative condition due to faulty nutrition.

embolus: a clot or plug, brought by the bloodstream, obstructing a vessel.

embryo: early developing stage of any organism.

endemic: prevalent in a particular region.

233

endocrine: pertaining to the ductless glands (hormonal)

endothelium: layer of cells lining the inner surface of blood-vessels and some body cavities

endophthalmitis: inflammation of the interior of the eye.

epithelium: tissue covering internal and external surfaces of the body.

exophthalmos: protrusion of globe, usually hormonal in origin.

extra-ocular muscles: muscles concerned in the movements of the globes.

filaria: a minute eel-like parasite

fibril: a minute filament

fornix: a vault-like space

gel: a colloid (jelly) of firm consistency.

haemoglobin: oxygen-carrying red pigment of the red blood cells.

hemianopia: absence of vision in one half of each retina.

herpes: a skin disease characterised by small clusters of vesicles (there are simple and Zoster forms).

hyphaema: blood in the anterior chamber.

hypopyon: pus in the anterior chamber.

intravenous: into or within a vein.

intraocular muscles: muscles serving the alteration in pupil size and focusing.

keratitis: any form of corneal inflammation.

lagophthalmos: inability to close lids together.

larva: immature stage in the life cycle of an insect in which it is quite unlike parent.

leukaemia: malignant disease of white-cell forming organs.

limbus (eye): the corneo-scleral junction.

metabolism: the sum of all the processes whereby the organism is able to live.

mucus: a slimy substance formed by certain (mucus) membranes.

neural: pertaining to the nerves.

new vessels: delicate, easily broken vascular fronds arising from definitive retinal vessels.

nystagmus: an involuntary rapid movement of both eyes.

nasal sinuses:cavities in the bones of the face communicating with the nose.

Glossary

occiput (occipital): the back part of the skull and the parts related to it.
oculist: ophthalmic physician or medically qualified surgeon.
oedema: the presence of an unusual quantity of fluid in specific sites.
oviduct: passage through which ova pass from the ovary to the womb.

pannus: a vascularized membrane spreading over the cornea.
parasite: an organism which lives upon another without contributing to its good.
pernicious anaemia: an anaemia due to failure to absorb vitamin B_{12}.
photocoagulation: cauterization of retinal lesions by use of xenon arc or laser beams.
proptosis: protrusion of the eyeball (non-endocrine causes).
plasma: the fluid portion of the blood in which the cells are suspended.
pus: a liquid product of inflammation formed mainly by white blood cells.
pole, posterior: the retina surrounding the macula bounded by the optic disc to the inner side and the superior and inferior temporal vessels above and below.

reflex, action: response of muscle and nerve to stimulus such as pain, cold, or pressure.

scotoma: a blind area in the visual field (often central).
siderosis: iron impregnation inside the eye following intra-ocular foreign body.
spondylitis: inflammation of the vertebrae (bones of spinal canal).
spermatozoon: male germ cell.
sulphonamide (sulphone): an antibacterial drug.
steroids: hormones from the adrenal cortex. Used as drugs in the eye mainly for their anti-inflammatory effects.

temporal: pertaining to the temple.
tendon: fibrous cord attaching muscle to bone.
thrombosis: intravascular clotting causing obstruction to blood flow.
toxin: poisonous substance.
thorax: part of body between neck and abdomen.
trauma: wound or injury.

vesicle: a small blister.
virus: the smallest type of disease-producing organism, responsible for many local and general diseases.

Index

Index

Index

ethambutol 29-30
eye, anatomy of 6-11
eyelids 82-3
    disorders 82-3
    structure and function 82
exercise 15
exudates
    hard 16
    macular 17

fibrosis, pre-retinal 61
field
    nasal 13
    temporal 13
    visual 13
finance for the blind 163-4
fissure, fetal 88
'floaters' 22, 37, 72
fluorescein
    angiography 16
    dye 16, 33, 65
foreign bodies 60
fornix, lower 66
fovea 13
fundus 9
    diseases of 19, 22, 25

galectocaemia 90
Galen 7
games 176
gentamicin 81
German measles 40
glaucoma 50-8, 106
    acute 57-8
    juvenile 89-90
    narrow-angle 55-7
    primary 52
        chronic simple 52-5
    secondary 25, 46-7, 52, 61, 64,
        88, 108
glioma 92-3
gonorrhoea 45, 80
government services 132-7, 158-
    61
grafts 35, 66
guide dogs 133, 155-8

haemorrhage 15
    retinal 16, 22, 25, 27-8, 96

subhyaloid 37
vitreous 15, 37, 64
'hammer and chisel' accident 60
Helmholtz, Hermann von 9
helping the blind 216-25
heredity 20
    and retinitis pigmentosa 20
herpes
    opthalmicus 83
    simplex 35, 45
    zoster 83-4
Hervé, St. 187
heterotropia 73
Hippocrates 6
history
    blindness in 115-18
    ophthalmology in 5-11
Hitoyasu, Prince of Japan 187-8
Homer 185-6
homonymous hemianopia 79
Huber, Francois 193-4
humour
    aqueous 7
    crystalline 6
    vitreous 7, 41
hypermetropia 69-73
hypertension 24
    ocular 54
hyphaema 36, 52, 63
hypopyon 27, 34, 36, 62

iatrogenic blindness 29-30
idoxuridine 34
infections 62, 94-6
inheritance
    dominant 20
    recessive 20
    sex-linked 20
injuries to the eye 59-68
    at birth 96
insulin 14, 16
International Agency for the Prevention
    of Blindness 213
international aid 214-15
international co-operation 210-
    15
International Council for the Education
    of the Visually Handicapped
    211-12

Index

Index

Index